EXPLAINING COLO

The Heartrending S

As told to
David Hooper

Dave Hooper

David Hooper

Published by
Chipmunkapublishing
PO Box 6872
Brentwood
Essex CM13 1ZT
United Kingdom

http://www.chipmunkapublishing.com

Edited by Steven Hoy

We would like to dedicate this book to our parents.

This is also for the millions of sufferers of mental illness around the world.

You are not alone!

Sue Kennedy and David Hooper.

EXPLAINING COLOURS TO A BLIND MAN

CONTENTS

EXPLAINING COLOURS TO A BLIND MAN

PROLOGUE

As we entered the flat, the first thing that hit us was the stench. It was overpowering. The fact that he had been dead for four days before they discovered him was obviously a major factor. However, it wasn't just that. The smell was ingrained into the very walls and floors and most particularly, the furniture. The chair that he died in was stained with years of filth and grime. On a table next to the chair, was the fish and chips that he had brought home, but didn't get a chance to eat.

The chair faced a wall, upon which was a large poster of a naked woman, which he evidently sat and looked at night after night. Underneath the chair and the bed were hundreds of porn magazines. The bed looked like it had never been changed, and the sheets and blankets looked like tea had been poured all over them. It almost certainly wasn't tea.

We picked our way gingerly through the detritus that covered the floor and moved into the kitchen. Piled from floor to ceiling were years and years worth of fish and chip wrappings and another pile of chocolate wrappings. It seemed that whenever he ate fish and chips and chocolate, (which it appeared he lived on), he kept all the wrappings. However, they weren't strewn haphazardly around the floor, but had been straightened out and put into neat piles.

The cooker was caked in grime, although not from use, as he never cooked. As far as we could tell, he lived on takeaways. There was one tin plate, one tin mug and one knife and fork.

We didn't spend much time in the bathroom. The bath was grimy and rusty through never being used. The toilet was covered in what I'm politely going to call filth. He had been taking medication for diarrhoea, the result of which was obvious for all to see.

Moving back into the bed-sitting room, we were about to get to work, going through the bags and bags of letters and documents that went back years. He never got rid of anything. Mum pointed to the wood panelled wall behind the chair, and said, 'Look at that wall. That's quite nice for a flat like this.'

On closer inspection, we discovered that it wasn't a wall at all. We slid it open to reveal row upon row of shelving, stacked with brand new clothes. From the labels, we could tell that they had been there for years, unopened.

Just then, the doorbell rang, so Dad went to answer it. When he opened the door, the woman standing on the other side almost fainted.

'Oh God,' she said, 'I thought you were a ghost. You're the image of Bernard. You must be his brother.'

'Yes that's right,' said Dad.

'I'm Mrs. Murphy. I live downstairs.'

'Come in,' said Dad. 'I'm Pat and this is my wife Doris, and these are my daughters Susan and Julie.'

'Pleased to meet you,' said Mrs. Murphy. 'I don't envy you the task you've got. He was a bit disorganised, wasn't he?'

'You could say that,' said Mum

'I used to do his washing for him', said Mrs Murphy, 'well, when he let me, at least. I would knock once a week to collect it, and often he would tell me that there was nothing. Then about once a month I would get a pair of underpants, if I was lucky.'

'You're very kind,' said Julie.

'Oh, it was nothing,' said Mrs. Murphy. 'He wasn't a bad old stick. He kept himself to himself. Anyway, I'll let you get on. Call me if you need anything.'

With that she went. Armed with rubber gloves and plastic aprons, we carried on sorting through the litter. In amongst the rubbish we found his Abbey National passbook with £20,000 in it. Then Dad moved a wardrobe, and found taped to the back of it, £10,000 worth of premium bonds. What a contrast. He had money in the bank, unopened clothes in his wardrobe, and yet lived like a tramp. I realised that I knew nothing of my uncle. I had never met him, and by all accounts, Dad hadn't seen him since they were young men, despite trying to contact him.

Bernard was Dad's half-brother and about ten years older. They shared the same father, but Bernard's mother died of flu during the First World War. Mum told me that Bernard and Dad didn't get on at home, and that Bernard was a pig to his stepmother. She told me that one day Bernard was particularly insulting to his stepmother and Dad snapped. He picked up a carving knife and chased Bernard out of the flat with it, threatening to stab him if he came back. He never came back.

Mum said that Bernard was similar to my grandad in nature. Grandad was not a coper and he hated change. One example was that he lived in a run down, squalid flat with damp running down the walls. It looked, by all accounts, like the 'Shelter' posters that you used to see in the 1970s. He was offered a nicely decorated and modern flat, literally opposite the dive he lived in, but he turned it down. He couldn't cope with moving even 50 yards. Mum said that when my grandma was dying in hospital, Grandad used to visit her, but refused to believe that there was anything wrong with her. He would shout, and berate her and tell her to pull herself together and get home to cook his tea. He was stubborn, belligerent and verbally abusive to his wife.

'A bit like Dad then.' I said

'Yes,' said Mum, 'very like your father.'

I knew that Dad's sister Eileen suffered similarly with depression and an inability to cope. She also spent time in a psychiatric hospital and had electric shock treatment. The pattern was emerging. As I looked around my uncle's flat, surrounded by the filth and grime, a shiver ran through me. Was I looking at my future? After all, I shared the same gene pool. I too have suffered from psychological illnesses for most of my life. Will I end up like this, I wondered. After all, I'm part of the same gene chain. I am my uncle's niece, my dad's daughter. Is it part of my genetic make up? Part nurture, part nature? Oh God, I hope not.

THE BEGINNING

I was born on the 27th of July 1959. It wasn't a very auspicious start. My mum's dad was being buried at the very moment that I was born. Mum suffered from post-natal depression, which was not surprising considering that her father had died just before my birth. She also had toxaemia and high blood pressure throughout the pregnancy, and as a result, I nearly died during the birth. The first few days of my life was spent in an incubator. My dad said I looked like a little angel, lying there like a little doll with perfect rosy features and golden curls. I won't say what my mum called me. I was told later that I screamed night and day for the first 18 months of my life. I've been a worry to them ever since.

I was quite an extrovert during my young life. I would memorize the stories that people read to me and when visitors came, I would pretend I was reading these stories from the book. I would recite them almost verbatim, using the pictures as my prompts. My aunts and uncles were quite impressed with my precociousness. I was a real con artist. I would also sing and dance in front of whoever happened to be there. I loved an audience.

I was also an incorrigible gossip. Whatever Mum and Dad said about people, I would dutifully pass on to everyone; including the subjects of the said gossip. In the end, Mum and Dad had to spell everything so that I wouldn't understand. I became a good speller.

I liked bedtime. My dad would sit on the

side of my bed and make up 'Piggy', 'Hedgehog' and 'Squirrel' stories. These were all characters he met on the way to work on his bike. I really loved these stories, and they carried on for a number of years, until I was about eight. I think my love of literature stems from this. This was before I 'bought' my sister.

For the first three and a half years of my life, I was the centre of the universe. Then one day my life was turned upside down when my mum told me I was going to have a little brother or sister. I would rather have had a guinea pig, but Mum was having none of it. However, she said that nothing in life was free and that I would have to pay for my new sibling. Blooming cheek. Not only was I going to get a mewling, smelly, baby getting all the attention, I was going to have to pay for it myself. Life's just not fair.

I started to save up all the golden pennies that Father Christmas and other people gave me. I kept asking if I had enough for a hamster, if I couldn't have a guinea pig. But no, for some reason they insisted on a baby. When I had enough golden pennies, Mum went away to buy the baby. In due course, Mum arrived back home with my 'purchase'.

I was left alone with this pink thing that I had bought. The pink bundle started crying. Ah, I thought, it's obviously hungry. I remembered we had some cakes and being the polite person that I was, decided to feed the visitor. The visitor didn't really appreciate this culinary feast and cried some more. On hearing the cacophony coming from this ungrateful guest, all the others came back into the room. On seeing what I had done, they all told me off. This was day one. I was the one in trouble and Julie was the good little angel whose mouth wouldn't melt butter.

This pattern was to follow me throughout my life. All I was trying to do was entertain our new visitor, but got in trouble doing it. I wouldn't have minded but the baby was obviously Chinese, or some other type of foreigner, as it couldn't understand anything anyone said and we certainly couldn't understand it. I told Mummy she should take it back and get a proper one. That didn't go down too well, either.

Mummy impressed upon me that I was to help her with this 'Chinese' baby. I never really learned by my mistakes though. One day Julie was lying there, crying. I remembered that when the baby cried Mum used to feed it and this shut it up. Right, I thought, she's hungry, I'll help Mum. I knew that Dad had Shredded Wheat for breakfast so it must be all right for Julie. I shoved a wedge of it in her mouth but although the crying stopped, so did the breathing. The pink bundle went bright red and Julie promptly grassed me up with a humungous scream. Mum came running in the room, saw what happened, and I got yet another smack. It wasn't fair. I was only trying to help.

Like the time Mum was boiling potatoes on the stove. She was upstairs at the time and I thought I would help her out by salting them for her. It wasn't my fault I couldn't read. Half a container of Ajax later and the potatoes were frothing nicely. When Mum came downstairs to see the broiling mess with the strong stench of ammonia she, not surprisingly, asked me what I had done. I proudly told her that I had helped her with the potatoes by salting them. She was not too impressed. Another smack on the legs. Meanwhile Julie was being fawned over as Miss Wonderful, but all she could do was eat, sleep, cry and smell. I was the one working my fingers to the bone, but was I appreciated? No.

One day, Mum took Julie and me out, and left Dad by himself. He asked Mum if he could do anything to help while she was gone. Mum thought about it and said yes, he could peel the potatoes ready for the evening meal. 'Ok' said Dad, 'I'll get right on it'. And so he did. He peeled every potato we had in the house. Every conceivable container held these potatoes. He had long since run out of pans, and so he utilised everything else he could get his hands on, including the washing up bowl. Mum came home with us to find the kitchen looking like the back room of a chippy. There were enough potatoes to feed an army.

'Patrick, what on earth do you think you're playing at?' asked Mum when she was able to speak.

'Well, you said peel some potatoes, so that's what I did', said Dad. 'You never said how many you wanted, so I did them all'.

We ate potatoes morning, noon and night for weeks to come, and Mum never asked Dad to peel any more for her again. Maybe that was Dad's plan.

During my early years I remember being Dad's little helper. We used to do things together, like shopping. Later in my childhood, being Dad's helper brought with it many problems. I had no idea then of the conditions which beleaguered him. I do now. I have inherited them, to some extent.

PRIMARY SCHOOL

My first school was Skyswood, which was directly opposite our house. I was quite happy and confident when I went there. In fact, where other children cried on their first day, I was laughing and told Mum that she could go. In fact, she was the one who cried.

My first teacher was Miss. Elliot. She was very nice, and I remember her as being quite bohemian, wearing Moses sandals and no tights. It's remarkable the things you remember as a child. That first year, I seem to remember, consisted mainly of playing in the sand pit or the Wendy house. I seemed to get on all right with the other children at that stage.

In my second year, my teacher was Miss Benson. I remember being given cards with words on to copy. Although I could do this, I didn't know what I was doing. I couldn't read but I could copy. I looked good doing it, but in hindsight, it was all a façade.

This phenomenon followed me into adult life. For example, I always came across well at interviews. I seemed a 'got together' type of person, in control, full of confidence. The truth was the opposite. From the age of about 11, when I went to Nicholas Breakspear, I had all my confidence knocked out of me due to bullying and other problems at home. However, I'll come that in a later chapter.

Back to Miss Benson and me with no knickers. Yes, even then I was attention seeking. I was in P.E class, doing head over heels on the floor, unaware of anything wrong. Miss Benson called me out and said 'Susan Kennedy, you haven't got any knickers on.' Story of my life. Anyway, they had spare knickers at the school just for such an emergency. Just for the children, I hasten to add, not the teachers, (although, you never know). I had to go home and tell my mum that I had no knickers on. She was a bit cross but also presumably, a bit embarrassed. Thoughts of the war effort flashed across her mind.

Another recollection I have in Miss Benson's class is the day I was nearly run over. Every afternoon, after school, Mum would come and meet me to help me across the road. This particular day she wasn't there. I decided to be helpful and cross the road myself. I looked left and right, as I had been taught, couldn't see anything coming and walked across. The purple Jaguar was on me in an instant. It stopped just short of me and I ran off screaming. The driver was in a rage and followed me to my house. I ran in through the back door while he was ringing the bell at the front door. I went haring into the dining room and hid under the table, petrified. The point is, metaphorically speaking, when I feel overwhelmed that's what I want to do now. I want to hide under the table. It's a throw back to my childhood. If I'm under the table, 'they' can't see me so 'they' can't get me. 'They' are whatever problems I'm having at the time. Be it dusting or hoovering or anything. Again, all will be revealed later in the book.

Another bad memory I have is of Louise Thornton's birthday party. Although I wasn't that friendly with her, for some reason I was invited. I think her mum was in charge of the guest list and I was a nice, polite, sensible girl. The trouble was, I was the only one. It was mayhem there. The children seemed to do exactly as they wanted. It just wasn't me. I was brought up in a quiet environment and was really out of my depth. I wanted to be anywhere other than there. This was the first time in my life that I had had these feelings. I was to have them regularly for the rest of my life.

I attended other similar parties where I felt out of my depth. I only really enjoyed parties that were structured and had an adult in charge. I felt safe in those settings. Having said that, there's always an exception to the rule. My sixth birthday party will remain burned into my memory for all time. I was allowed six guests, and they were all good friends of mine and all of a similar nature. We were enjoying ourselves as children do but Dad was trying to organise things as if it were a military operation. He couldn't cope at the best of times, but trying to cope with seven children was too much. In hindsight, I know that you shouldn't try to tell kids how to enjoy themselves. It should be spontaneous. My dad couldn't be spontaneous. Even the taking of a photo took ten minutes, with him arranging everyone like it was a royal portrait.

Of course, being the fiery redhead that I was, I had a strop. I felt that Dad was showing me up in front of all my friends. I had a miserable face, wouldn't cooperate with what he wanted and was critical of him. He finally had enough of me and chased me up the garden. When he caught me, he smacked my bottom hard until I cried, in front of all my friends. He then took me to my bedroom and locked me in. That was the end of my birthday party.

Looking back, that was the first time I had noticed my dad's temper when things didn't go right. It certainly wasn't the last time I would challenge him, although he never hit me again. Nevertheless, he certainly had rages that went on throughout our life when he would raise his fist to us. My fiery nature and his rigid outlook would often end in a major confrontation.

In September of that year, a catholic school opened two doors up from our house, St. John Fisher, so I transferred there. I hated it, and the standards were much higher than at Skyswood. I struggled in all subjects, including games, and came bottom in nearly every class. Most of the teachers were horrid and I spent a lot of my time thinking about ways of escaping this nightmare. I used to come home for dinner but I also remember going home one break time, telling the teacher that I had forgotten to take some medicine. All lies, of course.

My early view of life being wonderful was shattered. I lived for coming home or the summer holidays when I surrounded myself with a few choice friends with whom I felt safe. I always had a good imagination and was good at making up games and plays. In a way, I bought friendships by inventing these games to play.

One day I was sitting at the dining room table doing my homework. Dad had only just finished decorating the room. This was a mammoth task for him. He could never cope and built everything up to a high degree. In addition, he was a perfectionist, which is why it took him two years to complete. It was the equivalent to him of climbing a mountain. As I sat there, I couldn't get my fountain pen to work. I shook it vigorously and to my horror, watched as the ink flew out from the pen and stained the new wallpaper. When Mum came in and saw it, she went ashen. What would Dad say? I had ruined two years of worry, stress and anxiety in a second.

I decided to run away, and headed for the bus stop. Nothing came. I eventually came home and Mum kept Dad away from me for the next couple of days, although the atmosphere was palpable. That reaction of running away from my problems was to follow me throughout my life.

During this time, and throughout most of my schooldays, Dad had taken to running the local Mass centre, which was in St John Fisher's hall. I think the man that used to run it went on holiday one day and never came back. Dad took it on. I wish to God that he hadn't.

Dad has suffered all his life with what I now recognise as Obsessive Compulsive Personality Disorder. This is not the same as OCD, or obsessive-compulsive disorder, which many people have heard of. People with OCD experience tremendous anxiety related to specific preoccupations, which are perceived as threatening. They have to perform elaborate rituals to avoid or escape anxiety, for example, hand washing, or checking the doors are locked. These rituals have to be repeated in order to keep stress and anxiety at bay.

With OCPD, on the other hand, the person's dysfunctional personality produces anxiety, anguish and frustration. They are so deeply entrenched in their dysfunctional beliefs that they see their way of functioning as the 'correct' way. They tend to stress perfectionism above all else, and feel anxious when they perceive that things aren't 'right'. The anxiety is relentless, as everything must be precise, and the avoidance of error is of paramount importance. This perception produces procrastination and indecision. It could literally take up to 30 minutes to fill out a cheque, due to a rigid need to ensure that there are absolutely no mistakes. To make matters worse, they are reluctant to delegate tasks or to work with others unless they submit to exactly his or her way of doing things. Material is read and re-read until a sense of absolute clarity exists. Not only is it extremely time consuming, but the overall content of the story is lost. The forest is missed while examining each leaf, of each branch, of each tree.

For someone who is impaired by this illness, there tends to be an overwhelming need to be in control of his or her environment. Everything must be put back in precisely the correct place, otherwise control is lost. People suffering from illnesses like this can't control what's going on in their heads. Inside is all messed up; therefore, the outside environment must be as ordered as possible. Spouses can be subjected to daily scrutiny and given repeated negative feedback. Friendships (how ever long lasting they may be) are often fragile at best. Someone with Obsessive

Compulsive Personality Disorder, at the more extreme end of the range, project an air of anxiety and rigidity.

Often, being with someone with OCPD feels like walking in a field of land mines. One never knows when you're going to step on one and pay a heavy emotional price for crossing the rigid standards. Sufferers are preoccupied with details, rules, lists, order, organization, or schedules to the extent that the major point of the activity is lost. There are few moral grey areas for a person with OCPD; actions and beliefs are either completely right, or absolutely wrong. Their way is the correct way and all other options are 'WRONG'. Anger and contempt are rarely held at bay for those who disagree. When every decision seems to take on the same paramount importance and being correct is imperative, making even simple choices can become a nightmare. They tend to place a great deal of pressure on themselves and on others to make no mistakes. Exerting effort to contain 'out-bursts' of emotion is an everyday occurrence. The expression of anger tends to come out naturally and in excess.

That was my dad! That was why it took him so long to do the decorating. Of course, I didn't know he was ill at the time. To Julie and me, it was just Dad, and we did as we were told. Mum knew he was ill, but kept it from everyone, including us. My finding out about Dad's mental troubles, in later life, was crucial in understanding about my own problems.

Dad's OCPD was to manifest itself more prominently during his involvement at the Mass centre. This was because the Mass centre was very important to him, so the demands he put on himself were overwhelming. These problems would then be transferred to us, as we would have to help him. Helping Dad meant doing exactly what he said and having no say in how to do it, then taking the brunt if anything went wrong.

Every Saturday Julie and I would go with Dad to the Mass centre to place the chairs and dress the altar. This placement of chairs had to be precise, to the inch, in a perfect semi circle. The affect, if one were to look down upon it, would be like an auditorium. Dad would place the first few chairs, and Julie and I had to position the ones behind exactly.

Because Dad has never been fast to get going, quite often we would not even get to the Mass centre until after four. Consequently, we frequently wouldn't get finished until after 9pm. Mum used to encourage Dad to get there early to enable us to finish at a reasonable time. A row would then ensue, with Dad accusing Mum of being a nag. In the early days, Julie and I also helped Dad put the chairs away. He used to stay there after we did that, doing I don't know what, and came home hours later. Mum would be annoyed with him for getting in late when the dinner was ready, and yet another row developed.

A committee was formed to delegate the running of the Mass centre, as it was felt that Dad couldn't cope on his own. That much was true; however, he would never admit this. Nevertheless, when they dared to want different hymns from Dad, and had different ideas, it was too much for him. It was very much his way or no way. He had a blazing row with the committee and said that they could do it themselves. I think that came as a great relief for everyone concerned. It certainly was for the rest of us.

The Mass centre saga went on throughout my schooldays, and wasn't to finish until I went to college. Consequently, the troubles I had at school were compounded by the regime at home. This pattern was to continue throughout my life until I left home.

Before I move on to my Secondary school years, I should like to sum up my time in primary school. Although I was not popular at St John Fisher, I wasn't bullied there. I was just thought of as a bit of an oddity. I didn't like the school, but with hindsight, my time at St. John Fisher was a holiday camp compared with what was about to come. When I left, the headmaster, Mr. Higgins, confided in my dad that when he first met me he thought I was very intelligent and that I would be a high flyer. He said that he was very disappointed when I didn't accomplish this prophecy. I didn't achieve the required standard to get to Grammar School, and so was to go to Nicholas Breakspear.

Nicholas Breakspear was the local secondary modern school. In those days, secondary moderns were often looked down upon as somewhere for rejects. The high flyers went to grammar schools; the failures went to secondary modern. All I know is that Nicholas Breakspear had a very bad reputation, and hardly anyone came away with even a CSE, let alone an O level. The behaviour of the pupils was appalling, and the general opinion was that if you went to Nicholas

Breakspear, you were to be pitied, as there was little hope for you.

Mrs. Gettings, my teacher at John Fisher, took a few of us to see the school, before we were due to start. 'There you are', she said, 'not too bad, is it?'

'Besides', she said to me, 'you'll probably end up putting the wheels on Matchbox cars in a factory, if you're lucky.'

Her prediction was to come rather too close for comfort, later on in my life.

SECONDARY SCHOOL

If John Fisher was a bad dream, then Nicholas Breakspear was a nightmare. The bullying started even before I got to school. I lived a fair distance from the school, although just inside the 3 mile limit so didn't qualify for a free bus pass. There was a coach laid on by the school, although we had to pay for it.

The first problem was that no one told the coach drivers that they had to stop for us. We stood where we were supposed to, but invariably, they just drove straight past. When they did stop, the coach was almost full. No one would let me sit next to them; they would put their bags on empty seats or trip me up as I walked along the gangway. Meanwhile the driver would get irate waiting for me to sit down. The journey home was as bad. The drivers resented stopping at Marshalswick, as it was more work for them. Again, a seat was never made available to me.

On one occasion, the only vacant seat was at the back. This was where all the undesirables sat, smoking. I eventually managed to balance myself on the edge of a seat next to a boy called Paul Burke. He looked at me with a malevolent glare and snarled, 'What are you doing here? You're not wanted on this coach and you're not wanted at the school.'

This really cut me to the quick. To top it all, I had been prevented from getting off by the others. That was also a common occurrence. When I eventually got off the coach, I was very upset. Another girl, Janet Campbell, got off with me and offered to take me home. This girl was one of the bullies, but in my naïve way, I thought she was genuinely being nice to me. I took her to my house and we went round the back. I introduced her to my mum and said that Janet had helped me. Mum was very nice to her and as it was a hot day gave her a glass of lemonade. What I didn't realise until the next day was, it was all a set up.

The girl saw that we lived an old-fashioned way of life, and when we sat down to eat in the kitchen, she saw that the walls were yellow and patchy with ageing paint, and that the lino was worn and cracked. This was all relayed back to her mates at school. I was a laughing stock and ridiculed about things that I took for normal. My family was also ridiculed and this hurt me deeply.

The jobs around the house were done, not just in an old-fashioned way, but a very complex, precise and indeed, tortuous way. Take shoe cleaning. You would think, would you not, that cleaning shoes presents no problems? It's not something that you necessarily looked forward to, but nevertheless, nothing to get worked up about. Unless, that is, you lived in our house. Shoe cleaning used to last hours. For a start, nothing could begin until Dad got around to it. We wouldn't dare start without him; even scraping the mud off was forbidden and he would become extremely angry if we even suggested it. He was never fast getting going. Once he did get going, all the shoes that were going to be cleaned were placed in the garage where this mammoth task was about to take place. Each process, cleaning off the mud, applying the polish, cleaning off the polish and final buffing, was precise and specific and had to be followed exactly. This was Dad's O.C.P.D, but none of us recognised it in those days.

Another example was the weeding of the garden. Dad would spend hours on one spot getting every single hair of every weed out, then sift the soil until it was like graded flour. I must admit, the soil was fantastic once he had finished. The trouble was, the garden was so massive that by the time he had covered ten feet, the first bit started growing weeds again. On the rare occasions he let us assist him we had to do it in exactly the same way as him. It was all so mind numbingly tedious and boring. Dad couldn't cope with life, that's the truth, but he wouldn't let anyone else cope for him.

One day, Dad said he was going to be late home from work, so Mum tried to help him out by watering the garden for him. When he got home he was so incensed that Mum had the audacity to water the garden and was so convinced that she hadn't done it well enough, that he proceeded to do it again himself, for about four hours. He finally finished in the small hours of the morning.

That would happen with many things. We didn't dare do anything off our own bat or else there would be an almighty row. The paradox was, because Dad couldn't cope and everything took an age, all the jobs kept piling up. It was a no win situation. To this day, when I do a job, I'm always convinced that it hasn't been done well enough. If one hasn't spent hours doing a job then it surely can't be done right.

That first year at secondary school was probably the worst of my life. There wasn't a minute went by that I didn't hate it and I was constantly bullied. We had to queue outside the classrooms for each lesson. Everyone and I mean everyone, used to bully me there. I used avoidance tactics to get there as late as possible. They laughed at the way I looked, the clothes I wore, my hairstyle, everything.

When we got in the class, it was no better, as no one would let me sit next to them. I used to have to sit next to a girl called Moira, who used to wet herself and also stank. No one wanted to sit next to her either, which was why there was always a vacant chair.

When it came to books being given out, I was always missed. I had to go to the front of the class to get my own book, and invariably the teacher told me off for having left my seat. The teachers were useless and never spotted any bullying, or if they did, just ignored it.

The lunchtime queue was just as bad. Everyone I passed made comments and snide remarks about me. The older girls were especially bad, laughing at my shape. That was the beginning of my obsession with my stomach size and the precursor of my eating disorder. To this day, I am still unhappy with my shape. I was destroyed at that school and I have never recovered from it. I can't put into words the constant fear and dread I suffered for seven years. It was a living nightmare of terror and mental torment, where I dreaded every corner and what waited round it. The anticipation of what was going to happen next was probably the worst part. My body was constantly in a state of trepidation, the adrenaline pumping through my body ready for fight or flight. I never did fight. I never fought back. I just took it. The bullying hardly ever manifested itself physically. In a way, I would have preferred physical pain to mental pain. At least it would have been over quicker.

Going to the toilet brought with it its own set of problems. The girls wouldn't let me in, would trip me up and abuse me when they eventually did and then, when I got to a cubicle, they would look over the top and ridicule me some more. When I had finished they formed two columns that I had to walk through to get to a sink, where they would abuse me and scorn me even more. They made fun of my body, the way I walked and even the way I sounded while I was going to the toilet. This happened every single day. I would try to last until I got home to go to the toilet, putting off the inevitable for as long as possible.

P.E was the absolute low point at school. Not only was I not very good at it but it gave a lot of ammunition to the bullies. I hated undressing in front of the other girls. They constantly mocked the way I looked. I recall they used to wear all the fancy panties and I had on my sensible Marks and Spencer knickers. I was just coming up to the age of puberty and therefore highly sensitive and self-conscious about my body. I was developing more slowly than the other girls were, so that was remarked upon. Not that it mattered. I was ridiculed over the slightest thing. I was bullied because I was me.

They would hide my games kit so that I was late getting dressed. The P.E teacher was vicious. A tiny thing, but all muscle. Like all games teachers she was like a Sergeant Major, and was forever having a go at me for not being ready. I don't know why I didn't tell her about the things that were being done to me. I think that I was afraid, afraid that things would only get worse if I did. I was threatened on more than one occasion that if I told anyone what was going on, life wouldn't be worth living. Life wasn't worth living anyway, but I was still scared. They would take my towel and soak it in the shower so that I couldn't dry myself. They hid my clothes and trampled them into the mud. I always hoped that a teacher would see what was going on, but none did or if they did, they turned a blind eye.

Out on the games pitch, I had a terrible time. You had to stand in a line while the two captains would pick sides. Everyone was picked except Moira, the girl who stank, and me. It did my confidence a power of good to know I was the lowest of the low. Even when everyone else was picked and I was the only one left, I still was not wanted. The teacher had to force one of the captains, who vociferously complained, to have me and I would mildly amble on to the pitch, pretending that it did not matter. The other girls would then purposely miss the ball and relish hitting my ankles with their hockey sticks.

In later years I became rather good at cross-country running. This became an escape for me, as it was a solitary event and I could avoid all the bullies. I even started doing it during my lunch breaks, merely to avoid being near anyone and invoking yet more persecution.

Playtimes were also bad. No one played with me, not even the one friend that I had outside of school, Julie Latimer. She didn't play with me, not out of spite, but because if she had, she would have been bullied herself. Just to be seen with me was enough to evoke the wrath of these thugs.

I hated being around the football games as I had been hit on the head on numerous occasions by a football. So I used to go off by myself to an out of the way place. This was also my undoing as it was also out of the way for the bullies. The boys had football as their sport at playtime; the girls had me as theirs. They persistently used to surround me and torment me.

The anticipation was the worst part of it. Quite often, they didn't say anything; they just stared at me and prevented me from leaving. The expectation that something nasty was going to happen made me feel physically sick. Psychological bullying is far worse than physical, and the scars last much longer. In my case, all my life.

Because of the hellish life I was leading, I withdrew totally into my studies. I adored English and was completely absorbed in any book I read. This was the one escape I had. Because I had nothing else, I could concentrate fully on my schoolwork, and was getting constant 'A's and 'B's in most subjects, and at the half-year and end of year exams came top in my class. I also won the prize for the best exam results of the year at speech night. Of course, the Neanderthals in my class did not like this very much and one boy called Alan Doyle, said, 'Brainy people get brain tumours, so why can't Kennedy get a brain tumour and die'? The form teacher must have heard this remark but said nothing.

Even though I was top of the school, I didn't get to be head girl. I overheard a couple of teachers in the library say that I should be head girl really, as I had the top marks, but that they didn't think I would be suitable for the role, as I wasn't popular. They elected another girl instead, who happened to be one of the chief bullies.

I thought that by studying hard I would get to College and become a teacher, then I could look out for the vulnerable children, and help them. It was not to be though. The bullies would win in the end, as they usually do. Their hounding of me lives on in my mind to this day, as I never did become a teacher. I could never exorcise those horrific times and banish them to the past by helping other susceptible children. For this reason alone, I can never forgive those bastards who ruined my life.

It was not just being unable to become a teacher that was taken from me; it was any career, despite all the hard work and studying. All the work and effort I put in at school was to no avail. All I wanted to do in my life was to help people, especially those worse off than myself. However, due to the mental scaring and psychological damage done to me, there seems to be few people who have been worse off. It has taken all I have to get through life, let alone being able to help others. I hope those people from my school years are proud of themselves, and what they did.

Although I doubt if they remember any of it. It was just a laugh to them. I was in the wrong place at the wrong time. If it were not me, they would have found someone else to destroy. I hope nothing nasty happens to them!

At the end of the first year, there was a disco. As you can imagine, I did not want to go. Why would I want to have more of the same from the bullies after school hours? Nonetheless, Mum persuaded me to go. She said that if I went I might make some friends, as people would see me in a different light. I relented, but I insisted on having some new trousers to go in. I did not want to go in my school uniform, obviously. At that time, the early seventies, the fashion was trousers with a fringe on the bottom of the legs. I thought, in my innocence, that if I had the proper up-to-date clothes, I would be accepted.

Mum did not have much money for clothes. All our clothes came out of the family allowance. Dad was always on a low wage, so all his money went on the housekeeping. However, I kept on at Mum to get these trousers, as I would not go to the disco without them. She eventually relented, (I think Julie had to go without something), and we went to the shops. Mum insisted on one shop in particular. This was a good shop but dealt in mostly kids' clothes. I was almost a teenager and I knew that none of the girls from school would ever shop there. Nevertheless, that is where we had to go and we got my trousers. They had a little tassel around the bottoms and I thought I looked the bee's knees in them.

The day of the disco came and I went to school carrying my new trousers in a bag along with a bit of make up I managed to get. I knew the type of lipstick all the other girls used so I saved my pocket money, 1s 6p per week, for about a month and bought it. I also got an old eye shadow one of our neighbours was throwing away. At the end of the school day, I went into the toilets to change. I went into one of the cubicles so that no one could see me, put on my new trousers, did my hair, put on my lipstick and eye shadow. I did the best I could and did not think I looked too bad.

While I was in the cubicle, I did not realise that it had gone quiet. There were loads of girls outside, all getting ready. I should have known what was about to happen. As I opened the door, I saw dozens of girls in two rows, waiting for me to walk the gauntlet. They started humiliating me straight away, mocking my trousers, my make up, everything. They took my bag from me, which contained my school uniform and my make up, and tipped it on the floor. They threw my lipstick into the toilet and smashed the eye shadow against the wall. They then tossed the bag with my uniform in from one to the other.

It was horrendous. I cannot explain the utter humiliation I felt while they were throwing my bag back and forth to each other while I stood in the middle of them. I eventually got it back and I went to the hall where the disco was. It was awful. No one would speak to me. Decidedly, no one wanted to dance with me. I tried speaking to a few people but they all ignored me. Even Julie Latimer was too scared to be seen with me in case she was singled out.

I stood alone by the stage with a glass of orange juice in my hand pretending to be enjoying myself, but in truth, I was counting down the seconds to when I could go. I could not go home by myself, as I had no money. Julie Latimer's father was going to give us a lift home. Understandably, the enchantment of the trousers had worn off very quickly. It was not the trousers. It was the person wearing them. I was the easy target with whom these degenerates had their fun.

Even the mere mention of the names of these animals made me break out into a cold sweat; Mandy Almond, Ellen Kier, Maria Bishop, Eileen Oliver, Francis Flavin, Anne Southeran, Jean Walsh, Patsy Inglis, Irene Darg, to name a few. Names and faces that, to me, conjured up a nightmare. That nightmare remains with me to this day. Occasionally I have seen one or two in later years and the old fear and panic rises to the surface, even though I am a grown woman now. They did their job to such accomplishment that their handy work would live on forever.

During all this time, I tried to explain to Mum what was happening to me. It would have been easier to explain algebra to a baby. It was no use even trying to explain to Dad, he could not take anything out of the norm. It was much the same with Mum, really. She was too busy trying to run a home while coping with Dad. I did not have the vocabulary in those days that I have today, and I find it hard even now. If I said something like, 'The other kids don't like me, and they pick on me.

They won't let me join in'. Mum would say, 'Oh well, you just try and join in and go and make some friends'.

She was not being unconcerned; she just did not know the hell I was going through. She was always there for us, a hot meal when we got home, our clothes always washed and ironed. We were loved, but I felt unlovable because of what was happening at school. How can you explain mental cruelty? Although most of the bullying was verbal and psychological, I would rather it had been physical. You can explain a bruise or a black eye. Something could have been done about that. In those days, teachers would not become involved in what they would consider trifling things. If I had summoned up the courage and told them, the answer would have been to answer back and to get a shell on my back, give as good as I got. I could not give it back. It was not, and still is not, my nature. When the whole of the first year hated me, which was how it came across to me, how could I fight everyone?

One day the verbal abuse did become physical. I almost welcomed it. We had rural studies, which took place in an out-building of the school. As we were queuing to go in, one girl called Anne Southeran, kept on and on, goading me, 'Do you want a fight? Do you want a fight'? I ignored her as best as I could, but my stomach was all knotted up inside. She was a fat, ugly girl with blonde hair. She looked not unlike Miss Piggy. A teacher walked past us and told us to go into the classroom and that Mr. Nickerson would be along soon.

We went in and I took my place by the desk. With no teacher to supervise, the torment continued. The girl kept prodding and poking me, taunting me and pushing for a fight. Again, outwardly, I ignored her, but this made her even worse. She eventually snapped, grabbed my hair and pulled me to the floor. Before I knew what happened, she had me pinned down and started pummelling me. Her face and eyes projected utter hatred. The rest of the class crowded round and they all had the same look of loathing on their faces. The only kind words, if you can call them that, was from the boy called Alan Doyle, he of the brain tumour comment. He said, 'Let her get up. Don't pin her to the floor, make it a fair fight'.

It was hardly fair. I was punched and kicked not only by Anne, but also by everyone else. They stood on my fingers, spat at me, and were completely out of control. I thought I was going to die. It was just like the scene in Lord of the Flies, when Piggy is attacked. All the time they were hitting me I could see the look of repugnance on their faces. These loathsome creatures made me feel as though I was below contempt. I felt that I was a worthless human, insignificant and a waste of skin. To this day I think that I am unlovable and a waste of space. Well done everyone. You have ruined a human being's life.

Eventually Mr. Nickerson came into the room and broke up the fight. He shouted at everyone to get back to their seats. The fact that I was all battered, bruised, and cut and that I was surrounded by all the others did not seem to bother him. He treated everyone the same. No one was reported for it. The bullies had won again.

When I got home that night, Mum saw the state I was. She looked in horror at my dirty, torn clothes and all the bruising I had. At least she could understand what had happened to me this time. On the strength of this, Dad went to see the headmaster, Mr. Eastham, about getting me put into a different class. The head said that I would be moved at the end of the year to another form. He said that he could not make the other kids like me or talk to me. I did not mind not being talked to. I just wanted to be left alone.

Moving to another class gave me some let-up. I had one or two friends that I could stand next to in the playground. Although I still had to share other classes with the main protagonists, which was most of my year.

It wasn't just at school I was bullied, but outside as well. Two girls, Lena Killinger and Sandra Hooker, lived in my road. They didn't go to my school, so didn't know what was happening there. I must have come across to them as a victim. Maybe all victims are apparent to a bully. They used to prey on me and made fun of way I walked. In fact, they would do almost exactly the same things as the bullies at school. It was as if they had all gone to the same bullying academy. They would block my path and trip me up. They would make fun of the things I wore, how I looked, everything. It may not sound much now, but taken with what I was going through at school, I was in a very fragile state.

I avoided these two whenever I could, but that was easier said than done. I had to run errands for my mum to the shops so had to leave the house. I would walk the long way to the shops in the hopes of avoiding them. I used to go out earlier and earlier each week in order to avoid them. I was putting myself under immense pressure. They still found me, more often than not. I did try to tell Mum of these two, but she told me just to ignore them. 'So what if they're sarcastic about the way you walk', she said, 'rise above it'.

My home was becoming like a prison. It was like being agoraphobic, a condition I experienced later on in life. I used to dread outside jobs helping Dad, like apple picking or footing the ladder for painting the gutter, in case the Hooker or Killinger girls saw me. Let me explain. I had to foot the ladder for Dad while he picked the apples. They were painstakingly picked one at a time and handed to me. When we had a bucket load, they were to be sorted and lined up in the garage. I had to hold the bucket for Dad, as he had to be in charge of this lining up process. They had to be spaced an inch apart accurately, to within a micron. Of course, Julie or I could never be trusted with such a vital job. Our job was mostly holding things for Dad while he got round to doing his bit.

While all this orchard business was going on, we all had to be dressed the part. Dad looked like Frank Spencer, complete with mac and beret, and Julie and I looked no better, wearing old macs and Mum's old headscarves. Most of the time we just stood around like this doing nothing, (hoping not to be seen), while we waited for Dad to organize himself. The same thing happened when it was time for Dad to spray the trees; our important job was to hold the bucket in which the liquid was kept.

The cleaning and painting of the guttering was an even worse nightmare that gave an immense amount of ammunition to the Hooker/Killinger duo. Again, Julie and I had to foot the ladder for this task. Julie never seemed to mind these mundane tasks; she seemed to escape to her own little world, a practice that continues to this day. I, on the other hand, hated it. Once more, I had to wear the old mac and headscarf and look a complete nerd; (I would have liked the headscarf to cover my face). Apart from having to wait around for ages for Dad to get his act together, this job, which at the most should have taken a couple of weekends, took eighteen months. Eighteen monotonous months of living in fear of being seen by those awful girls; eighteen tedious months of complete and utter boredom footing a ladder; eighteen mind-numbing months of not being able to do anything else. I realise now it was not Dad's fault. It was his illness. Nevertheless, that didn't make my life any easier. I was living in hell at school and had no respite at home.

We tried not to wind Dad up or upset him in case he blew up. He did get angry with us from time to time, even threatening us with his fists. If anyone went against his OCPD problems, he just blew. You see, we didn't dare not to help Dad. We were required to 'assist' in whatever way Dad instructed. To refuse would incite a fury of immense proportions. Besides, Mum would plead,

'Do it for me. Do it for peace sake'. However, we got very little peace- especially internally.

Dad used to do the shopping and if he saw a bargain, he would get as much of it as was possible to carry. For instance, at one time we had 97 boxes of shredded wheat. 97! There were only four of us living in the house; how could we possibly eat all that before it went stale? Then there were dozens and dozens of toilet rolls, more than a mass outbreak of Dysentery would require. We also had rows and rows of jam. Dad arranged these in lines of Strawberry, Blackcurrant, Apricot, and raspberry, to be used in strict rotation. If it was a raspberry day and you deigned to pick strawberry, Dad would blow his top. We had to walk on eggshells all the time in order to keep the peace.

With Dad buying up the stockrooms of Tesco's, the spare room, (where everything was kept), quickly became full, as you can imagine. I have to explain that the lounge was uninhabitable for years. In fact, I was in my early twenties before we could use it. Dad took a long time getting round to things. In his mind, he had it all on his plate, (a saying he would chant like a mantra), and in a way, he did. He built things up to such an extent that everything seemed insurmountable. If you think that shoe cleaning took four hours, how long would decorating a room take? Everything had to be done to perfection or not at all, (the example of him being on his knees for hours at a time weeding a square foot of garden is a case in point); but obviously, perfection cannot be achieved. Therefore, he wouldn't even start a job for the fear of not doing it flawlessly.

He did try to decorate the lounge, but he never had much time weekdays, due to being late home most nights. Then on Saturdays and Sundays, it was the Mass centre. In between times, it was cutting the grass, weeding, shoe cleaning; the list goes on. He would never, ever, ask for nor accept any help, so the jobs did not get done.

He started on the lounge with a little pot of Polyfiller, going round and filling in the little hair line cracks. Week after week, this went on, until the walls were covered in little white lines. Really, he was procrastinating, as he was terrified of what he had to do. I can remember him shaking like a leaf before starting a job; his nerves were in such a state. I'm not belittling him here, he was not well and to some extent, I have inherited some of that illness.

To escape the horrors of my world, I used to lock myself in the bathroom every night and listen to the Capital Countdown. While the music was playing, I would rock back and forth imagining I was a 'normal' girl at a dance, enjoying myself, as I should have been. In reality, my mind was in torment. The sustained mental pressure was getting to me. The human mind can't take years of unrelenting pressure; furthermore, the adrenaline that continually surged through my body must have taken its toll. I think I used up all my future energy back then, just surviving; which in fact is what I do now.

Although I had a strong faith, I was even ridiculed for that. It was a Catholic school and so attending Mass was obligatory. I used to take Holy

Communion and was ridiculed by those who didn't take it. There was a statue of Our Lady in our school that I used to go and be near when I was feeling particularly vulnerable. I used to pray for her to help me, but of course, it seemed she never did.

THE SECOND YEAR.

The second year was marginally better than the first. Because I got good grades, I went up to the top set and therefore away from most of the bullies during lessons. Although I wasn't bullied as much, I was still not Miss Popular. I still crossed paths with them during playtimes and was bullied as much then. My friend, Julie Latimer, started sitting with me in class. One day the bullies got wind of this, got hold of Julie and locked her in the cupboard during lunchtime, in punishment for having the audacity to be my friend. She still sat with me after this, but sometimes even Julie would shun me and sit with someone else. Julie was luckier than I was in that she had other friends, whereas I would cling to her like a limpet. I did have a few others that I could stand next to in the playground, but I was always intimidated by the bullies, and that went on right throughout my school life.

Getting the school coach home was always a matter of making sure you were there on time, otherwise it would go without you. On one occasion, I was late getting to the coach as I had been rehearsing for the school play. Anyway, the coach had gone and I didn't have any money to get home, so I had to walk. It was a fair distance home, so I decided to take a shortcut through the grounds of Oakland's College. It was very quiet there and I was the only one about. Or so I thought. I heard a rustling in the bushes, and to my horror, a man emerged wearing a bra, suspenders and a girdle and was exposing himself. I was terrified. I ran off as fast as I could, looking round all the while in case he was following me. When I got home, far from getting sympathy and reassurance, I was told off for taking a short cut. The incident wasn't reported and for all I know, the man carried on what he was doing. I saw him again, from time to time, over the years. He was an alcoholic and an outpatient at Hill End Mental Hospital.

I mentioned before about missing the school coach due to over running rehearsals. This was for a play I was in, 'Love is the best remedy' by Molière. At first, I only had a small role and Julie Latimer had the leading female role. After a while, the drama teacher, Mr. Hoare, decided that I was better suited to the main part and Julie was relegated to a minor role. That caused problems with our friendship, and she went through a period of not wanting to sit with me. She was understandably jealous of me out-doing her, although we made up again later.

During my time in the play, from rehearsals to performance, I enjoyed myself immensely. I was working with older kids, and although they were not overly friendly towards me, they accepted me for the work I put in. I felt an immense sense of achievement and satisfaction doing this, and the play, and my part in it, had great reviews in the local paper. I think we performed it 3 times. My love of English was beginning to blossom and I felt at times that I 'belonged'.

I had another success in the second year. I liked cookery and was quite good at it. The Milk Marketing Board ran a competition with all the secondary schools in Hertfordshire. We had to devise a main course and pudding with milk as a main ingredient. Then we had to design a poster as part of an advertising campaign about why milk is good for you. All this was good news for me, as we could use the lunchtimes for working out our dishes and designing the posters, which meant I didn't have to be out in the playground where the bullies were.

Two girls from Hill Grove School in Hemel Hempstead came first and Barbara Ransom and I came second. She devised the pudding and I came up with the main course, which was a bacon roll in cheese sauce. We also got the prize for the best poster, which we collected at the Civic Centre. Once again, I got my name and photo in the local paper.

Staying on the culinary theme, every year at Christmas, each form used to prepare a hamper to go to deserving poor families. Many of these hampers would have been full of tins of baked beans, if the teachers hadn't intervened and shared them out with the slightly more worthy donations. One year a couple of the girls stole the bottles of drink that people had donated. There were some wonderful human beings at my school.

Paul Burke liked shooting things. That Christmas he shot a pigeon and brought it to school. That was to be his donation for the Christmas hamper. Later, one of the teachers told me how he had to dispose this pigeon very surreptitiously out of the mini bus window, so that the selected poor person didn't have to have roast pigeon for their Christmas dinner.

By the end of the school year, I was doing quite well academically. I won the History prize and the English prize, which also made the local paper. Notwithstanding my successes academically at school, I was still a bit of an outcast, an outsider, if you will. I was still bullied outside of school by the Hooker and Killinger girls, and that went on until I was in the fifth year, but by then the fear had set in. They only had to look at me to set off the panic. Even to this day, if I were to see one of them my stomach would churn.

The school also used Julie Latimer and me as a kind of recruitment advertisement at the primary schools. 'You too could go to Nicholas Breakspear and end up like these two model citizens', kind of thing. I wouldn't wish my time there on my worst enemy.

Overall, the second year at Nicholas Breakspear wasn't as bad as the first. There were many redeeming features about it. The bullies did not have so much access to me and I was achieving academically. Even so, all the bad things that happened in the first year, continued into the second.

THE THIRD YEAR

It was in the third year that the church youth club started. Mum and Dad encouraged me to go as they thought I would get on more by mixing with people. Mr. Barry, from the Mass centre, said that he would give me a lift. Unfortunately, the people I would be mixing with were the same ones that I had been avoiding at school. Since it was a catholic youth club, obviously many of the members were from my school, plus a few I didn't know. I had no friends there. It was absolutely awful from the start, even from standing in line to pay to get in.
One of the boys from my school, Paul Palmer, was standing behind me, showing off to the others, simulating having sex with me, then pulling a face and saying, 'Oh no, can you imagine ?' I was there with my best dress on and it was as if I was back again in the first year. I was ridiculed; no one would dance with me, so I stood at the back by the wall hating every minute of it.

I used to go and wait by the phone box at the end of the road for most of the evening, waiting for the time to pass when Mr. Barry would come to pick me up. I wanted to leave, but Mum and Dad made me go, saying that I wouldn't make friends if I didn't mix. I did want to make friends but every time I tried, I was rebutted. Julie Latimer went occasionally, so it wasn't so bad. At least I had someone I could stand next to and with whom I could talk.

My whole experience of it was dreadful. All the boys wanted to do was spray Coca Cola everywhere and fight each other. I think I went there for about eighteen months, and then gave up completely. I couldn't stand it anymore. I would have stopped going earlier, but I always had a desire to get out of the rut I was in and better myself, but maybe it did more harm than good.

One day, during the summer, Julie Latimer and I were at the bottom of the school playing fields. We went there as the thugs couldn't be bothered to walk that far to bully us and we got some peace. However, on this occasion Jean Walsh and Patsy Inglis were down where we were. While I was making a name for myself as an academic achiever, these two were making a name for themselves as thugs and bullies; I therefore avoided them as much as possible.

On this day, they called Julie and me over to them. They pointed to the other side of the hedge where a man with his trousers round his ankles was exposing himself. I must have been a magnet for these men. They couldn't report it as they wouldn't be believed, (being the habitual liars that they were), so it was down to Julie and me to report it to the headmaster who contacted the police.

When the police came, I had to make a statement. Mr. Eastham asked me to describe what I saw in my own words. Well, the only word I knew was 'Willy'. I didn't know what else you called it. I'm sure they must have known what I saw; it certainly wasn't a turnip, or anything. Anyway, they caught the man. Again, he was a patient who had escaped from the mental hospital.

Mr. Eastham brought me home, along with the police, and explained everything to Mum and Dad. I don't think they were very happy about it. Not because of my ordeal, but because they didn't like people to see our house as it wasn't decorated, and it interfered with everything they had to do. The police showed me a book of photos of suspects, but I hadn't really taken much notice of his face, I was too busy looking at his turnip. This second exposure reinforced my fear of men. My only experiences of men up to that point had been the boys at my school humiliating and rejecting me, and those two men exposing themselves to me.

One of the brighter points of the third year had been my involvement in the school play. That year it was Romeo and Juliet, and I played Lady Capulet. This was a much more arduous play and a lot more demanding than the one from the previous year. I enjoyed doing it but it was taking up too much of my time and my schoolwork was suffering as a result. My French teacher, Mr. Betts, suggested I gave my thespian skills up and concentrated on my academic work, which I subsequently did. Whereas I enjoyed the rehearsals for the play, there was a social side of which I wasn't too keen. For example, everyone involved in the production was taken to Stratford to see a play and, while I wasn't bullied or excluded or anything, I still felt a bit of an outsider. Most of the other people involved were older than I was and therefore they stayed with their peers.

In July of that year, I was to go to France with my cousin John and his wife Anne. I was very much looking forward to this, as I had never been abroad before. We were to stay at a house in Elne near Perpignan, which belonged to Anne's sister. I stayed over in John and Anne's house in England, and met Sylvie there, (who was Anne's niece and was about my age), who had been staying with them on holiday. The next day, we all drove over to France.

I didn't really enjoy the holiday at all, as I was very homesick. Anne was cold and unfriendly towards me, and she spoke a lot of the time in French, which I didn't understand, and stirred up a lot of hostility against me. At the time, I couldn't understand why she was so against me and so intimidating. Sometimes I could hear her and John rowing about it. I heard John say, 'She's only a kid, give her a break'.

Since then, I've learned from several people that Anne was jealous, and therefore hostile, towards people to whom John was close. I have been told that she was the same with Norah, John's mum.

I also didn't like a lot of the food. A fish stew, with the eyes of shrimps floating on top, springs to mind. Anne's mother made it, and Anne said it was the height of rudeness to refuse to eat it. Another time, we went up in the mountains for a week in a place called Réal. We stayed at Anne's Grandparent's cottage. One day we had to go out and catch frogs. We were going to have frog's legs for dinner the next day. I was given the job of holding the bag, in which the live frogs were carried. While I was walking along, I could feel the frogs jumping up to try to get out of the bag. I hated that feeling. I let the frogs out of the sack and they escaped. Meanwhile, a farmer had killed a milking lamb, so we were to eat that instead. Yippee! They also had some snails that they kept in a fish tank. They were fed on Thyme, which purifies them. Snails, like lobsters, are cooked live. They were put on the grill and cooked then everyone got a pin and you had to pick out the flesh from the shell. Not surprisingly, I didn't want any of this. Again, Anne lost her temper with me so I had to eat them. I felt sick.

One day we all went to a dance. I felt very nervous about going, but I put my best dress on, one that my mum had bought me especially for my holiday. John made me take it off as he said it looked too formal for the occasion, which put yet another dent in my confidence. The dance took place in the village square, out in the open. A man asked me to dance with him but I think Anne put him up to it. I was pleased as I was usually left at the side like a wallflower. However, this man started groping me, and of course, I wasn't used to that. I looked over to the side for some support, and I could see Anne laughing. She might have thought that it was all a bit of fun, but I felt very uncomfortable. She said later that she wanted to see me get drunk and dance on a table.

As you can imagine, I was very happy to get home. It was my birthday while I was away, and one of the presents I got when I arrived home, was 'Welcome Home' by Peters and Lee. That broke my heart. While I was away, my R.E teacher had left a bible and some material for my O level in R.E. I immersed myself in this homework to blot out real life.

Although Mum and Dad never had much money, they always made sure we had a week's holiday somewhere, even though a lot of the time I'm sure we would have been better staying at home. Dad found most of our holidays in the Dalton's Weekly, in the cheapest section. It certainly wasn't much of a break for Mum, as most of the places we stayed at needed a good clean before we could even start the holiday. Moreover, it was all self-catering so Mum just carried on as if she were at home.

Dad, on the other hand, wasn't interested in helping Mum clean the place or even help to unpack; what Dad was interested in was where he could get some mature cheddar cheese and crusty rolls. This was his first and only priority. No one else would dare go and get it. He insisted, and of course, for peace sake, no one said anything.

It wasn't much fun for Julie and me either. Being two young girls on holiday all we wanted to do was to get to the beach. However, Dad was just as slow on holiday as he was at home; he used to spend ages in the bathroom. Only when he was finished, was everybody else allowed a turn. Then he would go down to the shop to get what was needed for the day and Mum would have to prepare it for the picnic. We got to the beach about lunchtime. I'm not criticising Dad here. He was sick, (I recognise it more now than I did at the time) and he couldn't cope. He couldn't cope with life and he certainly couldn't cope with holidays. The way he did survive is the way he has always survived, with obsessive-compulsive behaviour and rituals. He would create behaviour patterns and routines with which he had to adhere. Left to his own devices he could endure life; however, if there was one tiny fly in the ointment, he would explode with rage.

Dad had to work late the night before our holiday to catch up on the work he should have finished. This meant him finally getting in the bath in the small hours of the morning and Mum not getting any help with the packing. Well, when it came to unpacking the suitcase at the other end, it transpired that Mum had forgotten the alarm clock. Dad completely lost his temper because of Mum's error. Obviously, it was all Mum's fault; she should have remembered to pack it. After all, didn't Dad 'have it all on his plate'?

She went out and bought Dad a new alarm clock out of her meagre housekeeping money, as an anniversary present, just to keep the peace. Why he needed an alarm clock, I don't know. He never rushed.

Dad taught me to swim. Most kids are happy with that achievement. I remember being extremely embarrassed. I have always been terrified of water, so it wasn't easy for me. Anyway, we all went to the swimming pool and Dad took me in the three-foot bit. What a sight I must have looked, with my swimming hat and water wings. He made everyone get out of the way while he held me; (I was about six foot at the time.) My arms and legs were flailing about while he shouted to the whole of the assembled audience, 'Look Doris, look

Hilda, she's doing it, she's doing it, she can swim without me holding her'. Meanwhile Mum and Aunty Hilda were pretending it wasn't them he was addressing.

Another embarrassing time was playing 'Ball O on the beach'. For a start, Julie and I had to wear swimming hats, even though the most we were going to do was paddle. You had to stand in a certain spot and Dad would throw the ball to me then I would throw the ball to Julie, she would throw it to Dad. But it was Dad who decided who would throw it to whom. He didn't like it if you threw to someone else for the hell of it. Once I had reached fourteen I naturally didn't want play Ball O on the beach. However, Dad got angry, saying that I was spoiling the holiday for everyone, and Mum asked me to do it 'for peace sake', so I carried on until I was nineteen, playing Ball O on the beach, with a swimming hat on my head.

When we were younger, we went on holiday by train or bus, with Uncle Bert sometimes taking us. However, after countless driving lessons and about twelve driving tests Dad got a driving licence. He bought a rep's car from work. It was a white two door Marina, which had had the life bashed out of it and was in a terrible state and the boot was filled with sand, for some reason. The passenger door did open, but if you gave someone a lift, you had to work the door for him or her. You had to lift it up first as it had dropped down on its hinge.

The first holiday we took in the car was to Westgate. Dad and I had to do a couple of dummy runs first for part of the journey. We didn't do many as, of course, Dad had too much else on his plate. The planning of the journey was like a military operation. We couldn't go on any major roads, (motorways were a complete no-no), and so we had to plan the journey using all minor roads; even if this meant going miles out of our way, which it invariably did. I was the map-reader of the group, which if you knew my map reading skills, would give you an insight into the others abilities.

Dad was in a terrible state of nerves. Mum, Julie and Aunty Hilda sat in the back and I sat in the front with Dad. We left home about six in the morning to avoid as much traffic as possible. He used to hate people racing and wanting to overtake us. Couldn't they wait; after all, we were doing 20mph! 'Let them maniacs wrap themselves around a lamp post' was one of his favourite sayings.

After a while, our car started making funny noises and kangaroo jumping, not unusual when Dad was driving, but this time it wasn't Dad. We got as far as Harlow when the car finally sputtered to a halt and gave up the ghost. Dad would panic at the slightest thing, so you can imagine the state he was in now. Luckily, there was a garage directly opposite where we broke down and we managed somehow to get the car in.

The mechanic looked at it, sucked through his teeth, and told us that it could be fixed but that we would have to leave it there. Well, when we used to go on holiday by train, we only took what we could carry. Because we had a car for the first time it was loaded to the gunnels. All our clothes and toiletries had to come out, and we had even packed food, which we couldn't leave. So off we trudged, loaded down like sherpas, to the nearest bus stop.

We got home that Saturday afternoon, hoping no one would see us and waited for the phone call to say that the car was ready. We had to wait until the following Tuesday as the Monday was a bank holiday. 'Uncle' Ron, our next-door neighbour, took us as far as the bus stop in town and then we had to get two busses to get back to Harlow, weighed down again with two hundredweight of clothes. We finally got to our holiday destination Tuesday night. We had to come home the following Saturday as we only had a weeks holiday. Was it worth it, I wonder?

We didn't have a lot of luck with holiday accommodation wherever we went. One holiday flat we had was the upstairs of a woman's house, with no door separating us. The woman who owned the flat had a son who had had a nervous breakdown and was forever just wandering up to where we were staying, and kept calm by cutting the buttons off the sofa. We hoped that there were enough buttons to last the holiday. We didn't like to think what he would cut off next.

Another place was so filthy that it would need demolishing before it could be condemned. It needed cleaning from top to bottom. Dad didn't seem to worry about it too much. We were there; he had paid, so that was that. We found an old, antiquated vacuum cleaner in a cupboard and tried to get up the worst with that. Unfortunately, it blew rather than sucked and made the place even worse than it had been.

The woman that owned the place had one eye, and had a daschund that also only had one eye. Perhaps together they could see in stereo. Mum tried to talk to this woman, but she would not answer the door. When we eventually did confront her, all she said was, 'Well, you've paid for it so you can take it or leave it, I don't care'. Dad wouldn't leave. He just blew. That was our only holiday and he couldn't really afford that. Therefore, to make the most of it, we had to go out and buy plastic cutlery and paper plates just so that we could have something clean to eat off. Not that we wanted to eat there, but we couldn't afford to eat out.

Aunty Hilda always used to come with us on holiday, otherwise she would have never gone away, but on this occasion she would have been better staying home. She had been given the box room, which had no windows, had filthy sheets, (like the other rooms), and was a breeding ground for the neighbourhood's spider colony. There were huge great beasts in there, and consequently they made their webs during the night. Hilda had to part these webs like curtains every morning.

We christened this place The Parrot House, as the woman owned a parrot and the seeds it was eating and indeed its droppings, used to come through the floorboards from the flat above, and we would find ourselves covered in it the next morning. I can't say that this was the happiest holiday I have ever been on.

On reflection, I can't really say I had ever been happy on family holidays. I used to watch other girls of my age and envy them. They went out at night to dances or the cinema with boyfriends and they certainly had more freedom than Julie and I. I knew that I would never have a boyfriend of my own. I could never have that life. I was too repulsive, a reject. I can remember being very depressed about this. I never had a young life.

THE FOURTH AND FIFTH YEARS

Towards the end of the fourth year, my English teacher, Mrs. Bongers, decided to put me in for O level English Language a year early, which I passed. At the end of the fifth year, I took the rest of my O levels. Because the teachers were not sure whether I would pass all the subjects, I was also to take them at CSE level. The idea was that if I failed at O level, I would probably get the CSEs. The unfortunate thing was that the syllabuses for the O level subjects were completely different to the syllabuses for the CSEs. Therefore, I had to do twice the work for what would be just one pass. I achieved O levels in Literature, History, Cookery, Religious Studies and Geography, and CSE grade 1 in French. In addition, I got CSE in needlework, and maths. Naturally, I was very pleased with these results and so were Mum and Dad. Not only did I get the O level prizes on speech night, I also received the English prize once more.

The daughter of one of our neighbour's, Fiona Hudson, was having her 16th birthday party. I was invited purely because I was a neighbour and of a similar age. We weren't really friends and she wasn't my type, although we played together a bit when we were younger. I didn't know anyone else there, as Fiona went to a different school than me and consequently had invited all her school chums. Many of Fiona's friends were of the same ilk as the yobs from my school. She wasn't like them, but apparently used to mix with them. She used to go along with whatever they wanted.

One of the games they played involved going into the kitchen and kissing a boy. When it came to my turn, I couldn't go along with it. I was terrified of boys anyway, and these were really rough types. They had made fun of me throughout the party and I couldn't wait to get away. I eventually made an excuse and started to leave. These horrible girls followed me out, circled me, and told me to kiss one of the boys. Naturally, I refused and they ridiculed me, called me names, and said that I was frigid. It brought back all the bad memories of the first year when I was surrounded and derided. I finally got home, shaken and upset. Once more, my hope of socialising and making new friends ended in disaster.

Before going into the sixth form, we had to do work experience. I went to do mine in a bank with two other girls. My idea was that although I had my heart set on being a teacher, if I didn't pass my A levels, I could perhaps get a job in a bank. However, I found it boring. I decided to concentrate on my A levels.

THE SIXTH FORM

The two years in the sixth form were my happiest at school, and in some respects, the happiest times of my life. I was still withdrawn as far as social occasions went, although I did have a few like-minded friends around me who were taking the same courses as me. I felt comfortable with this little group, which gave me some confidence.

Another happy time during this period was my Saturday job at Norbury's, which was the local greengrocers. It was a very busy shop and I had to keep a running total in my head whilst talking to the customers. The time used to fly past. Some very nice people worked with me, including Joan, the manageress, and Mr. and Mrs. Norbury, who worked there on a Saturday morning. In addition, a very good-looking boy called Phillip Avery worked there. I was very interested in him, but he was about three years older than I was and, anyway, was already involved with someone. Not that I would have made my interest known to him. As far as I was concerned, I wasn't worth looking at. Why would he be interested in me? Wasn't I beneath contempt? I had been told that I was often enough.

The teacher we had at the start for the A level course was Mrs. Bongers. I liked her very much, although she was very bohemian and absent minded. Unfortunately, she had a breakdown and couldn't carry on teaching. Julie Latimer and I put a lot of work in on our own, but finding where we could study was an art in itself. There wasn't a sixth form common room, so we had to use corners of the library. When the library was full, we had to find alternative places. Sometimes we found an unused classroom, which we could use, but sometimes we had to make do with what was no more than a cupboard.

Because of the effort we put in, it was understandable that we were annoyed when the new teacher, Mrs. Johnson, wanted to change our syllabus. She wanted to teach the books she had studied at college. Obviously, that would make life easier for her, as she didn't want to learn what we were studying. She was a rubbish teacher anyway, being only interested in flirting with the male members of staff. We had a meeting with the headmaster, and Julie and I spoke vehemently about this change. Mr. Eastham agreed with our argument. He could see how hard we had studied, (which was a rarity in our school), so in order for us to continue with our syllabus, he had to recruit some new teachers.

Mrs. Thring was an Oxbridge graduate, and came initially to the school to teach us. She was an excellent teacher, but my favourite was Sister Loretto. She was a wonderful person and superb teacher. In fact, they both were, and both brought the subject to life for us.

In October 1976, we went with Mrs. Thring and her family to the Lake District for a holiday, to study further the Lake poets. This was the best holiday that I had ever had. We went to the places Wordsworth, DeQuincy and Coleridge had written about. Mrs. Thring was very proper and precise and I felt very comfortable with her and safe. Apart from this break in the Lake District, I missed out on any other social activities. All my time away from school was spent studying, apart from my Saturday job at Norbury's. Most of my peers at school had involvements outside of school with boyfriends and parties, but I concentrated on my work. I had to study hard as I wasn't a naturally quick learner. There were boys that I fancied in the sixth form, but I was too nervous to act on it. I feared rejection and humiliation.

Joanna Norbury invited me to her engagement party. I didn't really want to go, due to my experiences at other similar functions. However, Soraya, a neighbour of ours with whom I was friendly, wanted to go. Her father made the proviso that she could go as long as I went with her. As Soraya was keen, I went for her sake. Up until then, the only parties I had gone to were the neighbours Christmas and New Year events. I was all right at those because it was mostly adults, and Mum, Dad, and Julie were there. Luckily, there were older people at Joanna's party, those who worked at the shop and their friends. Consequently, it wasn't all youngsters. My strategy, therefore, was to stick to the older guests, like Joan, who was the manager.

While I was hobnobbing with these people, my charge, Soraya, was slowly but surely getting drunk. She had been knocking back Bacardi all night. Somebody called me up to the bathroom where I found her sitting on the edge of the bath, having been violently sick. I was in a panic now. There was the person I was supposed to be looking after, completely paralytic. What was I going to do when her strict Turkish father came to pick us up? We got a lot of coffee into her, and she seemed to sober up enough to get into her Dad's car unaided. I don't know if he ever found out.

I was put in for the R.E exam in the January of my final year. The idea being that if I failed, I could take it again in the summer. If I passed, then I could concentrate on my English studies. I found it hard to study both subjects. By now, I was finding it harder and harder to take stress and pressure. I was not to realise it at the time, but my nerves were shot through from the sustained trauma at school. The pattern of my future life was beginning to unfold.

I passed the A level with a grade B. Mr. Eastham came round our house to tell us the news personally. I was the first person at my school to get a grade B in R.E. I could now concentrate fully on getting my English A level. The norm at our school, and indeed I suspect most schools, was to enter three A levels. I knew that I couldn't cope with three, so Julie and I managed to get out of the third one. We were also supposed to do games, but we got out of that as well and just concentrated on our studies.

My life was my studying. I worked hard at school and then when I came home in the evening I would have my tea and go to my room. I allowed myself until 6pm to listen to the radio. It was during this time that I would daydream and imagine myself as a social satellite and enjoying myself. This was my escape. All my contemporaries had proper boyfriends and went to dances and parties. I had my imagination. From

6pm until about 10pm, I would study solidly. I was extremely focused and determined to pass and to become a teacher so that I could help other vulnerable children like myself. I didn't realise at the time that I was heading for a fall.

After taking the exams, it seemed like a huge part of my life was missing. Indeed, it was, but on hindsight it affected me more than usual. One day I went to the launderette with Dad and felt a wave of blackness descend over. I felt as if life wasn't worth living, and I was in a pit of despair. I didn't recognise the symptoms of depression then. However, I would recognise them more and more as my life went on.

Although I got a B grade A level in English, (which was the highest grade anyone from my school had achieved), I didn't achieve my qualifications with ease, and I had to work harder than I had ever worked to attain them. The oppressive life I had lived helped to concentrate my mind. Now I was to leave school and move on to college. How would I cope there?

I had already been for the interview at Digby Stuart Teachers Training College in Roehampton, earlier in the year. At the time, I wanted to do a three-year certificate course in teaching, and then either use that certificate to get a placement, or carry on an extra year and convert it to a degree. The very day that I went for the interview, all colleges, including Digby Stuart, stopped doing certificate courses. Therefore I would have to do a full degree course if I wanted to teach. I was to study for a B.A in English and Religious Studies.

I was terrified about going away to Digby. I was to be one of only two girls from a Secondary Modern school. All the others were from grammar schools or private schools. I would be a fish out of water, especially with all my bad experiences of times away from home. The fact that I had led an insular and protected life meant that I would be very vulnerable.

My last few days at home before going off to college was spent in the back garden scything the grass on the back lawns. I know what you're thinking. Most people use a lawnmower. The fact is, Dad had put off cutting the grass for so long, that it was almost up to my waist. I was half expecting to find a Japanese soldier from the Second World War, waiting to surrender to me.

On the evening before I left for college, I had tea with the family and watched a bit of T.V. That evening, as I prepared to go out into the world on my own, was the last time I would eat normally, it was the last time I was not to have a problem around food, and in fact, it was the last time that I was fully free from depression, and all the other problems that went with it.

I wanted an early night to prepare myself for leaving for Digby in the morning. I was completely unprepared for life away from home. I had led a sheltered, protected life, up until then. My early night idea came to nothing. Dad decided that now was the time to tell me about bank accounts, as I would need one now. He only had six weeks to tell me, but as with everything Dad did, he left it until the last minute. It didn't help my nerves at all.

FROM UNIVERSITY TO THE BENEFIT OFFICE

The day finally arrived for me to leave the nest, so to speak, and go out into the world by myself. That was quite a daunting prospect for one as naïve as me. Mum, Dad and Julie all travelled up with me to Digby Stuart in Roehampton, and when we got there, I looked around for a girl I had met when I had my interview. I quite liked her, so when she suggested that we shared a room, I readily agreed. Unfortunately, I couldn't find her, but another girl, Jane, attached herself to me and asked me if I would like to share with her. She looked a bit down at heel, a bit like me really, and Mum liked her, so I agreed. Big mistake.

Jane was from a private school, and was one of five children from a military family. The parents brought all the children up as if they were in the army. She was very hard and selfish, and very go-ahead. She was good at everything she did, and I just wilted in her presence. If I got up in the morning and found Jane's clothes soaking in the sink, instead of bothering her, I would go and wash in the communal washrooms. This was a major problem for me as I still got very anxious about communal places and corridors. I kept reliving the bad experiences I'd had at school.

There was only one desk in the room, so Jane used it. I found somewhere else to work; it was in a block called East. At the very top, in the unheated attic, was where I did my studying. Jane was never horrible to me or bullied me, it was just that she was a very dominating character, and I was very easily intimidated; in fact, I still am.

We were responsible for cleaning our own rooms. I remember that there were big balls of fluff floating round the room, which were a product of the central heating system. There was also a thick layer of dust all around the room, and we had no cleaning materials to deal with it. This was my first experience of having a fear of dust. It continues to this day.

My food problem also started while I was at Digby. We had all our meals laid on; a cooked breakfast if you wanted it, a big mid day meal, afternoon tea and an evening meal. No one would ever starve there. Many of the girls would miss at least some of these meals, but Mum and Dad encouraged me to eat them as they had all been paid for. I ate the meals, but I would also binge eat in my room to try to stem my unhappiness. I would eat anything, chocolates, biscuits and cakes, anything I could get my hands on. I hadn't learned in those days to eat without getting fat. My family are all built like greyhounds, we're naturally slim, but I was gaining weight rapidly. I weighed about ten stone, which is the most I have ever been.

Although I wasn't being bullied any more, and I had a few friends at Digby, I was desperately unhappy there. The damage had already been done. During my school years, I just couldn't cope with any pressure whatsoever and the pressure was just getting worse. Some of it I put upon myself. I really wanted to be a teacher, but subconsciously, I knew that my dream was becoming unattainable.

I went back to Nicholas Breakspear in the November of that year to receive my A level certificates and the Canon Keanan cup. The school awarded this each year to the person that had tried the hardest. I saw all my contemporaries there who were collecting their A levels. They all said how well they were doing in their respective careers, while I was wondering what was happening to me. Why wasn't I happy?

I also went back at Christmas for the school disco. I wanted to prove to myself that I could go; that I could turn up as one of the successes, without fear. All the school bullies had left by this time and I was a woman at University studying to be a teacher. Little did anyone know.

I started at college with the intention of doing a B.A, with a teaching certificate at the end, but I changed my course for a B.Ed, in drama with a teaching course. I then changed again for a B.Ed in English, and then finally I changed one more time to a B.Ed in religious studies. All this chopping and changing was because I couldn't settle in and felt out of my depth. I thought, wrongly, that if I changed courses I might meet someone in harmony with me and that it would all become easier. However, I was fooling myself. I shouldn't really have been there at all. With hindsight, I should have just used my A levels and gone out to find a suitable career. None of this moving about was helping me, as whenever I changed courses I had a lot of catching up to do, which put me under even more pressure.

I was so lonely and unhappy at Digby. From the minute my family left me on that first day I felt lost. I had never lived on my own except of course times away on holiday. I had never even done my own washing before. Even when I was at school and living a life of hell, at least I had the haven of going home at night, albeit to an overprotective existence.

There was a phone box opposite Digby, and I was forever phoning Mum. We never had a phone at home at the time, so I used to arrange a time for Mum to be in our neighbour Evelyn's house and rang her there. I tried to convey to Mum about my unhappiness at Digby, and my struggles just to cope with living there, never mind trying to study. However, I didn't have the words to put across how I was feeling and I don't think Mum ever really understood.

I was able to come home occasionally at the weekend, and it was wonderful when I did. On one visit home, I took a shortcut through Skyswood school grounds. When I got to the gate, I saw Mum standing at our front door. Unfortunately, the school gate was locked. In a way, my looking at Mum through a locked gate was how I felt about my life; that I could see normality through the bars, but that I was locked behind them and I couldn't escape. Even now, I still use the analogy of looking through a plate glass window at normal life and wonder how I can get to the other side.

I still had quite a strong faith in those days and used to spend long evenings in the chapel at Digby on my knees praying for help. I didn't know what was happening to me, but realised that I was very low, very unhappy and unable to cope. Although I desperately wanted to be a teacher, I knew that I was not motivated enough to carry on. I desperately needed help and sought it through my religion. I didn't realise it at the time, but I was at the beginning stages of a breakdown.

There was a medical centre at Digby and one day I went in, ostensibly about an in-growing toenail. While I was there, I told the doctor about my feeling tired all the time and my lack of motivation. He diagnosed depression, which was the first of many times in my life that this diagnosis would be made. He put me on two types of medication; I think they were called Montipress and Motival. They were the old style of anti-depressants and are not available today. They were both sedating drugs, which only added to my problems; in fact, these drugs sedated me so much that I nearly fell in front of a tube train one day. The doctor also sent me to a psychologist at The Tavistock Centre in London to try to help me cope. I had two or three sessions there, which didn't really help. I was to find out through countless future sessions, nothing ever really helped.

If I stayed at Digby at the weekend, I would sometimes go to the village church in Roehampton, as life in the college was like living in a goldfish bowl. One day they asked if anyone would be able to help as a Sunday school teacher at the convent there. I volunteered and went along with a nun that lived in the convent. I enjoyed this time, and I remember walking through the kitchens and watching the novice nuns working there. I loved the peacefulness of it all, and I envied them their serenity. It reminded me of home and brought back memories of Mum doing the cooking in a warm kitchen. My homesickness came to the fore once again.

One of the nicest people I met at Digby was Sister Bridget Macken. She was a student there, studying to be a teacher of R.E. and History. I spent many happy afternoons in her rooms at Digby. She had a cardboard box that she used as a coffee table, and we used to sit there together to study. However, my illness had started to take over now so I found it very hard to concentrate, even in those tranquil surroundings. Nevertheless, I enjoyed my times with Sister Bridget, and we still keep in touch to this day.

By some miracle, it seems to me, I passed all of my first year exams; in fact, I got the top marks in my college. I don't know how I managed it, as my illness was progressively getting worse. I went to see the Dean, Miss Bradbury, and she said that I needed a break from study and suggested I had a sabbatical. The idea was that I would have a year off, then I would be refreshed enough to continue. I didn't know it at the time, but I would never return.

The first part of that sabbatical year, I did nothing. In a way that just made matters worse. I don't know if Mum and Dad really understood what was happening to me. I'm sure they didn't know about all my problems, especially the food related ones. My binge eating continued during this time, although my control of it had improved in as much as I now ate things that would not increase my weight, for example All Bran. I would eat a box a day. I would still eat the meals Mum made, as one never refused the food Mum put in front us. However, one of the other discoveries I made at this time was the effect of laxatives. I had started on the slippery slope of Anorexia.

After a while of being at home, word got around that I was there, and Mr. Norbury came round to see me. He said that Joan, the manageress, was taking a long leave of absence and asked if I would like to fill in for her. Thinking of the happy times that I had when I was a Saturday girl, I went back part time. Of course, it wasn't the same. Things never are when you go back. For a start, I wasn't a Saturday girl anymore; I should have been getting my degree so that I could become a teacher. I felt ashamed. People were obviously interested to know why I was there and not at college, but what could I tell them? I was too humiliated to tell them the truth, which was that I couldn't cope with it. I felt that they wouldn't understand and why should I tell them anyway? Also weekdays were never as busy as Saturdays, so there was a lot of time spent standing around; time to be questioned some more; time, also, for me to reflect.

During that year, we had a classic holiday on the Isle of Wight. We drove there, which again, was a big effort for Dad. I went with Dad for another dummy run for that holiday. I seem to remember going via High Wycombe. Anyway, on the day, we did find our way to Portsmouth for the ferry, but when it was our turn to board the boat Dad couldn't get the car into the parking bay. He was going forwards an inch, going backwards and inch, back and forth, back and forth, almost wearing a rut into the deck, with Mum and Aunty Hilda pretending they were with someone else. In the end, one of the ferrymen told Dad to get out and he parked the car for us. Parking has never been one of Dad's strong points. Even on an empty road, it would take him ages to line the wheels up precisely six inches from the curb.

When we got to our holiday flat, Mum, Hilda and Julie carried the luggage in, leaving me to guide Dad to a parking spot. Back and forth, back and forth, as usual, and finally, after twenty minutes, he was in. I breathed a sigh of relief and leant against a tree.

Well, I didn't know my own strength. The tree started bending at an alarming rate. 'That's it,' said Dad, 'we can't park here; the tree will fall on the car'.

As a result, we had to go and find another empty road to park in, (about two and a half miles from our digs). Once Dad parked, that was it. We never went anywhere else in the car. We travelled everywhere by bus.

I was very depressed on this holiday, and one day I was making up the beds with Aunty Hilda and I just broke down and sobbed and sobbed. I was so tired that I couldn't do anything. What struck me was that Mum and Dad just carried on as if nothing was amiss. I don't think they really understood what was wrong with me; they certainly didn't recognise that I was having a breakdown.

The journey home form the Isle of Wight was a replay of the journey there. We left our accommodation at four o'clock in the morning to beat the traffic. Of course, we had the ferry to drive on to. This was as bad, if not worse, as the first attempt. We nearly ended up in the water. Back and forth, back and forth, inch by inch, Dad just could not park the car. Eventually, one of the ferry workers more or less dragged Dad out of the car and parked it himself. However, Dad took so long messing about that the ferry actually missed its departure slot. All this did nothing to help how I was feeling at the time.

Back home and I was still working at Norbury's, and still hating it. I had applied for a job at Stevenson's, who sold school uniforms and expensive children's clothes. Now, at that time I had to go into hospital to have all my wisdom teeth removed. This was a blessing in disguise, as it gave me the opportunity to leave Norbury's. As with everything to do with me, it wasn't so simple. My teeth were very badly impacted and embedded into the jawbone. By all accounts, this was quite a major operation. I think that they had to break the bone to remove these teeth. After having this operation, I was in agony. My face had swollen up like a balloon, and had turned all colours of the rainbow. I knew how bad I looked when Dad and Julie came to visit me. The look of horror on Julie's face said it all. I was due to start at Stevenson's a week after my operation, but I was so ill that I had to delay it for three weeks. I think my physical condition may have hampered my recovery, as I was taking laxatives regularly now and was nowhere near the ten stone that I was at college.

I eventually did start at Stevenson's, but I was not happy there. I thought that I would be working in the school uniform section, but instead they put me into the expensive clothes department. This was dead during the week, as most of the sales were on a Saturday. Therefore, there was nothing to do all day, apart from dusting the odd model and sweeping up, hardly my favourite occupation at the best of times. In fact, the highlight of the day was the coffee break, which just about sums it up.

After work, I had to wait ages outside the shop for Dad to pick me up. He was never on time. Ever! Julie or I would never dare to catch a bus or walk home if Dad was going to pick us up or there would be a blow up. None of this helped me with regard to my health. I had obviously had a breakdown. I couldn't cope with life, I had no motivation nor incentive, my memory was going and I felt very low.

After a boring day at Stevenson's, all I wanted to do was go home. I could do without waiting outside the shop for Dad. The worst part was standing there, seeing people that I knew, and hiding from them in case they asked me any questions. One day I saw Michael Corey, who was the boy at Nicholas Breakspear that equalled me in academic achievements. He was walking along full of confidence carrying an attaché case, obviously getting on in life and using his brain. What had my life become? What was I doing with my brain? To say that life was unfair would be an understatement, a thought that would stay with me all my life.

In the August of that year, I handed in my notice at Stevenson's. I was still telling myself that I was going back to Digby in September, and told the manager of Stevenson's that I wanted a month off before going back to do a bit of studying at home. The truth was that when I got home, I didn't go out again. I had developed agoraphobia. I couldn't even go as far as our front garden. I was still able to 'help' Dad, footing ladders and holding things for interminable lengths of time, and I could go out in the car so I was able to go to church with the family.

I also used to go with Dad when he filled the car up with petrol. What a performance that was. I think the only reason that I went with him, was that everyone else had refused. Whenever Dad filled up with petrol, he would go and pay and then he would sit in the car and fill in a book with details of how much petrol he had put in, how many miles he had driven since the last time and any other irrelevancy he could think of. All this took ages, while the queue of cars behind got longer and longer; with the drivers calling Dad all manor of colourful names with the accompanying hand gestures. Dad was oblivious to all this, and when I did draw his attention to it he would just say, 'Let them wait, haven't they got any patience?'

When asked why he did it he would just blow. You never questioned Dad as to why he did anything. I heard him saying one day that he did it to see if he had a petrol leak. I would have thought the empty tank and smell of petrol might have been a clue, but there you are. You can't change Dad.

Dad came up to me one day and told me that he had worked out why I got ill in college. 'I've been thinking', he said. 'I've been trying to work out what you have been doing differently at college to what you did at home'.

'Oh yes', I said, wondering what on Earth was going to come next. 'What?'

'Well,' he said, 'when you were at home you had Shreddies for breakfast everyday. You told me that you couldn't get them at college. Do you think that's what has caused you to be ill? Not having Shreddies?'

I don't remember what I said to that. I got used to the strange things Dad would come out with. One thing I do know though, you never argued with Dad. If you told him he was just being daft, he would blow. I didn't have the energy to argue.

Mum got me to venture out a bit at a time to try to overcome my agoraphobia. I would start by just going to the bottom of the drive and back. Then it would be to the next-door neighbour's house and back, then further and further. The start date back for the next year a Digby was looming, and I was determined that I was going back to finish my course and become a teacher. I made myself walk to Fleetville, which is a suburb of St Albans. I only got half way when I saw a group of boys coming towards me. I just froze in sheer panic. All the old fears and worries came back to me.

When I got home in floods of tears, Mum said, 'Well, if you can't even walk to Fleetville, there's no way you can go back to college'. I knew that she was right. I phoned the Dean of studies at Digby Stuart and told her that I would be unable to return. I could hardly speak through my tears. She was very nice to me and told me not to worry, that I might be able to return later to resume my studies. I knew deep down that it was never to be. I knew that my dream was over, all my plans were shattered and that I would never fulfil my ambition to become a teacher. The feeling of being a failure, of letting down my family, and myself, has never left me.

Mum tried to help my cleaning phobia by giving me jobs to do around the house, for example dusting and hoovering. Mum was very particular about cleaning, and everything had to be done perfectly. I spent hours dusting rungs of chairs and underneath the sideboard. She asked me to vacuum the dining room carpet. This carpet had a pattern of squares on it, and I was on my hands and knees, because I didn't have the strength to stand up, hoovering a square at a time. I really hated this and I would dread doing it. I know that Mum meant well, but it was doing my illness no good. In fact, if anything, it made me worse.

In later years, when life became a round of counselling sessions, the various psychologists, psychiatrists and mental health professionals all said the same thing; that Mum making me do the housework when I was going through a very vulnerable time was the worst thing that could have happened to me. It made me associate cleaning with depression, fatigue, and a feeling of being overwhelmed.

It wasn't Mum's fault. She thought that she was helping me, but even her philosophy of 'You have to achieve every day to feel good about yourself', only made me feel worse about myself; I thought I must be lazy for not wanting to do it. I still think that of myself. I had years of watching Dad doing a job, any job, and having it take him hours, weeks or even years. It had to be absolutely perfect. Added to the fact that Mum's standards were very high, made everything I did seem sub-standard.

I still build things up in my mind, as I don't think that I will be able to do them properly, which makes my depression worse. My dad is similar except that, to overcome his fear of doing jobs, he would put them off for as long as possible by doing other non-essential tasks, (for example the painstaking weeding). He always told Mum that he didn't have time to decorate because I was ill. He 'had it all on his plate' because he had to cope with me. I have come to understand a lot about my dad's illness, as I have inherited it to a degree. I think, in a way, Dad was relieved that he had something, or someone, on which to blame his own shortcomings. He certainly would never admit that he was ill.

Every week I scanned the local paper, to see if there were any jobs available. I knew that I had to have a job, but I also knew that there was very little that I could cope with, (apart from the fact that I wasn't qualified for much). I applied for various posts but, as I thought, I was unable to do any of them.

Around this time, I went to live with my Aunty Hilda. I felt that I needed a bit of space from the regime at home. While I was there, I got a job at the Colindale Job Centre. Unfortunately, I only lasted there a week. I hated the job, as my illness meant that I couldn't cope with the pressure and the learning I had to do. Added to that, living with Hilda wasn't really helping me. She was used to living alone, and so had her own way of doing things. I didn't feel I could relax. There were certain restrictions that I had to adhere to, including only being able to use a certain amount of toilet paper and only being able to flush the chain a certain way. I could understand where she was coming from. She had an old toilet system and was frightened of it breaking and that she wouldn't be able to afford to get it fixed.

I decided that I'd had enough. What I did next will haunt me for the rest of my life. I went in to the Job Centre, and rather than be honest and tell them that I was ill and couldn't cope, I told them that my mum was ill with cancer, and that I had to go home to look after her. Of course, all the staff were very sympathetic and consoling and everyone was very nice. I left the job, but I have never forgiven myself for what I said. The guilt will live with me forever. When I got back to Hilda's, I told her that they had laid me off, as they didn't need me. I lied to everyone, in a vain effort to cover up my illness. I realise now that I should have been honest with everyone.

I went back home to Mum and Dad's, as I realised that living with Hilda didn't really help me. In all honesty, I didn't know what would help me. My illness was getting progressively worse. I was still suffering from agoraphobia, my anorexia was as bad as ever and my energy levels had hit rock bottom. I was tired all the time and I had no motivation to do anything. I was severely depressed and I felt that life wasn't worth living. What was I to do? I thought that I had better do something, rather than just sit in a chair all day. I decided to go out into the garden to do some weeding. I hated weeding at the best of times, especially the way Dad wanted it done. Nevertheless, it was something that I could do. Or so I thought.

I was on my hands and knees with a little hand fork, and not even having the energy to use it. Aunty Hilda had come round that day and saw me in the garden. I looked like I had just been released from a concentration camp. She was shocked at the sight and told Mum that something had to be done about me, and that I had to see a doctor right away. I think that Mum and Dad had put it off, as they didn't want to admit I was mentally ill. Mental illness had a stigma about it in those days, and in fact, it still does. My parents, especially my dad, are of the kind that, if you ignore a problem, it would go away. My problem would never go away.

I went to see my G.P. He was very nice and seemed to understand my problems. He gave me a prescription straight away for my various symptoms, and that started a life time of medication; some drugs were better than others, all had their own side effects, but nothing ever really worked. I’m still hoping for a miracle drug to this day.

David Hooper

FROM THE BENEFIT OFFICE TO THE CONVENT

I have always had a drive, an inner strength, to better myself. I think I inherited this from my mum. Because of my illness, this has not always been a good thing. If you don't set yourself challenges, you can't fail. On the other hand, I have never been a quitter. I could never just sit down and do nothing for the rest of my life. Although failure has dogged me all my life, if I were to have given up altogether, my life would have been over. It is only this inner strength that has kept me going, and similarly, it's what has kept my mum going, as well.

In the February of 1980, I decided I had to get a job. I looked through the local paper to see if there was anything I could cope with. Despite my A levels and a foundation course at college, I was not qualified to do anything. Most jobs required secretarial skills of one sort or another, and I had none of these. However, one advert was for a temp job in the Civil Service. I enquired about this and was told that the Luton Unemployment Benefit Office was recruiting, and would I like to go along the next day for an interview. To give them their due, my parents, especially Mum, were very wary of me working in a benefit office. She thought I wouldn't be able to cope. Her prediction was to come true, but at the time, I was frustrated with sitting about at home. I needed to be doing something, to become a human being again.

It was a Herculean task to get to Luton, as my agoraphobia was still affecting me. However, I did make it and arrived for my interview. The place was a complete dump, and I should have seen the warning signs. This was 1980 and the Thatcher era was in full swing. There were redundancies everywhere, so the benefit office had never been busier. They were desperate for help. I could almost have been wheeled in inside a coffin, to be taken on. They did interview me, but never asked any incisive questions. Basically, name, address, do you want to work here? Right, start tomorrow. It really was as quick as that.

What training I had was abysmal, and I was placed straight on the front counter. At first it wasn't too bad, as I was on fresh claims. All I had to do was take the details from the people who were claiming for the first time. The work was quite repetitive but seemingly never ending. The queue would stretch out of the door. Maggie Thatcher had done wonders for ordinary working men and women. NOT!

I worked with a lady called Thelma, who was quite motherly towards me and helped me, so I was quite protected. Most of the other people in the benefit office, on the other hand, were quite rough. It seems they really did take anyone on. Many of these people would get drunk during the course of the day. After a while of working there myself, I found that I couldn't really blame them.

One woman, Wendy, got friendly with one of the Personal Issue claimants. These were people with no fixed address, and would be given a personal issue Giro cheque over the counter. After a couple of months of going with this down and out, Wendy was an alcoholic, and had put on masses of weight. Eventually, after not turning up for work, she was sacked; even the benefit office had some standards. She then became a client on the other side of the counter claiming a personal issue Giro herself, as she too had no fixed address by then.

It was a dire place, and everyone was subjected to all kinds of abuse and threats, both verbal and physical. I worked on the fresh claims counter for six months, after which I was sent for an interview in London and was told I could stay on as a permanent employee. As a permanent employee, they wanted me to be able to do all aspects of the work. They especially wanted me to work on the general enquiries counter. Again, the training for this was laughable, not that I had a sense of humour by that time.

At that time, Vauxhall's were laying off hundreds of staff and the queue of claimants went round the block. I wasn't adequately trained for this job and was bluffing most of the time. The counter I worked on was equipped with a Perspex screen, to protect one from the claimants. This was designed not to shatter under force, but to fall in as a whole. To some of these people who had had their life shattered by Margaret Thatcher, I was the face of authority. It was my fault that they were unemployed, my fault that they couldn't pay their bills, my fault that they had five screaming kids, in fact my fault for everything under the Sun up to and including the hole in the ozone layer. When the rage took over these people, they went for me, via the Perspex shield, by which time the police had to be called. This happened to me on numerous occasions. You got no help from the management. They were all useless, couldn't cope with the pressure and didn't want to be there themselves.

Thursday was Personal Issue day; when all the down and outs without any fixed address would come in and get their Giros. They nearly all had drink/drug problems and they all smelt. They would come in and urinate and defecate in the office. You can imagine the smell. We always had trouble with them, and even if they got their Giro, they would swear at you and say that it wasn't enough and how could they buy a flagon of cider with that? There was always trouble at some time during the day, so we usually called the police out on a Thursday.

Often, we had mothers leaving their children with us, saying that they couldn't cope any more, so we had to get Social Services in to take them away. I also had numerous threats to the effect that people were going to follow me after I left work and would beat me up. I don't know if any of them did follow me, but the threat was enough. It was back to the school bullies and the Hooker/Killinger duo. I was forever looking over my shoulder, just waiting for something to happen. Like at school, the waiting was the worst part.

During my lunch hour, when I had the strength, I used to go to a church in Luton town called Our Lady Help of Christians, and attend the lunchtime Mass. I desperately needed some help and I would beg God to give me some freedom from the hell I was living in. I felt that the more I prayed, the more chance there was that God would relieve some of the agony I was going through.

By this stage, my life was spiralling out of control. I had no social life to speak of and my time at the Benefit Office was horrendous. The only control I had was in food. I could control my food intake if nothing else, which is how all anorexics start. I drastically restricted what I ate, and each day I took to work a small bag of All-Bran, which I would pick at during the day. I couldn't sustain this discipline and every now and then would have a massive binge. This was not a binge in most people's eyes though. For example, I would eat a block of jelly. This would expand in my stomach and I wouldn't be able to eat anything else.

Of course, I lost a lot of weight, and my Doctor referred me to a psychologist at Hill End Hospital, called Dr. Compton. This woman was quite strange, (I was later to find out that most Mental Health Professionals were quite strange), and was a born again Christian. She felt that by praying over me she could cure me. How many times would I hear that in my life? It was during these sessions with this Doctor that I found out that my home life was not normal and that my father was very sick. My illness, I was told, was a combination of nurture and nature. This revelation brought out a lot of anger within me. How dare my dad have given me this unbearable life, this debilitating illness that has stopped any potential in me? I blamed him for stopping me from doing any good, from achieving my goal in life and causing me so much pain and suffering.

I don't blame him now, of course. That would be like blaming a parent for passing on a rogue gene that they didn't even know existed. I know he didn't pass his illness on to me deliberately. He has tried all his life to do his best for us. He loved us, we loved him, and I still do love him. He has many, many good points, and it is sad that people have to suffer as he has. He just should not have had children; apart from the illness that he passed on, he just wasn't able to cope. Later on in life, I was advised not to have children myself, as I would pass on the self same illness.

My weight continued to drop at an alarming rate. At my lowest, I weighed five stone twelve. That was a very perilous time for me. My stick-like legs hardly had the strength to carry me up the stairs at work. When Dr. Compton saw me, she said that I had to go into Hill End Hospital because I was a danger to myself. I didn't like the idea of going into hospital, so I promised her that I would not lose any more weight. The truth was that I couldn't sustain the harsh regime under which I had put myself. Therefore, I did start putting on weight a bit at a time.

At work, I was moved once more to another department. This was across the road, and I had to work with an awful woman called Gwen, who was a complete bitch to me; in fact everyone who worked there were ghastly. My job was to fill in the blanks in standard letters: names, addresses and dates when people's benefits were suspended. I did hundreds of these, day in and day out. This was mind numbingly boring, but if I were honest, I wasn't able to cope with anything else. I hated this place and counted down the minutes as to when I could go home. It was like being at Stevenson's all over again, including having to wait at St. Albans train station for hours, for Dad to give me a lift home.

At home I would try to eat as little tea as possible, and what I did eat I would try to get rid of with laxatives. The fatigue was extreme, I looked like a concentration camp victim, and the depression was black. I would drag myself up stairs to bed only to be woken what seemed like five minutes later by Mum, for another day of hell.

I had no social life to speak of while I was working at the benefit office. I was forced to go to a couple of Christmas parties while I was there, but I hated them. They mostly consisted of people getting drunk and flirting with each other. People used to come back so drunk that at first we took them for Personal Issue claimants. In fact, one man was so drunk he had actually turned green. I had never seen this before, I thought it was just a saying, but he was doing quite a good impersonation of Mr. Spock.

I didn't really have any friends and in fact, when I had my twenty first birthday party, the guests were Mum and Dad, Aunty Hilda, Aunty Nora and Uncle Bert. There was no one else I could invite. To rectify my sad social life, I contacted Sister Loretto from Nicholas Breakspear. I was always very fond of her and I think that I was really trying to recapture my happy time in the sixth form. The look of shock on her face when she saw me said it all.

She understood the importance of me having a social life and making some friends, but knew of my fear of socialising. She introduced me to a local church group, which lead to me finding a

London based group called the Westminster Missionaries. As a result, I met Dana, Andy and Ita, who became close friends. I now had a social life, albeit consisting mainly of bible readings and discussions, but that was ok because I could handle that.

Meanwhile, at the benefit office, we got a new manager, a Mrs. Thatcher type, who had been drafted in to whip us into shape. She found out about my illness, and the fact that I was seeing a psychologist one afternoon a week. In order not to upset her and possibly lose my job, I agreed to use my half day a week at the clinic as my annual leave. This was my holiday, half a day a week seeing a psychologist. I had no other time off in two and a half years.

Meanwhile, Dad was having his own trouble at work. Although he did the job perfectly, he would check and re check everything, and therefore only get a fraction of the work done that he should have. He used to have extended lunch breaks in order that he could do the shopping. He then had to stay late at night to finish the work he should have done during the day. He was eventually made redundant in February 1981. This was a very hard time for my dad, and by association, the rest of us, especially Mum. It is hard enough for anyone when they're made redundant, but when you're ill, it is doubly tough.

Dad scoured the local papers looking for suitable vacancies, although he was never fast at doing this. Every advert was scrutinised minutely, as he was really trying to find an exact replica of his old job. The Friday adverts were eventually replied to on the following Tuesday. Needless to say, they were all long gone. Any encouragement from Mum for Dad to get a move on in applying for these jobs just ended in a blazing row. This was the early eighties and unemployment was rife. You had to apply for any vacancy swiftly, or it would be gone. Employers could pick and choose who they took on. Office work was now completely different to what Dad was used to. Computers were now the 'in' thing. Dad didn't have a clue about them, and so was not even in the running for the most basic clerk's job. Another factor going against him was his age. He was in his late fifties, and the thinking in those days was that at that age, you were past it.

Coming off the phone, having been knocked back yet again from another prospective employer, was very distressing for Dad. He would sit at the kitchen table with Mum and go through the whole conversation, blow by blow, trying to analyse what went wrong. He broke down in tears, when the humiliation finally got to him. He found it degrading that we had to survive on his unemployment benefit plus my wage. Although he never earned much, he was always the breadwinner, and a very proud man.

Occasionally though, Dad would get past the first hurdle, and receive an application form through the post. This would take him an age to fill in, (as he wouldn't allow anyone to help), but he would also add extra pages telling his prospective employer all about the rising cost of living, and how much Persil cost, or his life story, all of which was totally irrelevant to the job application. He rarely got to interview stage. By the time the form got to the relevant personnel department, the job was long gone.

To keep himself busy, Dad took on all the shopping. Wednesdays and Fridays were shopping days. This would take the whole day, as it involved going to every shop and market stall to get the bargains. This was the only way he could make ends meet, as he only had his meagre unemployment benefit plus what I earned to live on. We had no savings. Meanwhile, Mum said to Dad, 'While you're looking for work, you can use the rest of your time gainfully by decorating the lounge'. The lounge was unused from the day Mum and Dad moved in, and never decorated. Dad was forever going to 'get around to it'.

Reluctantly, Dad agreed, and so began a long, drawn out process of painting and papering. Right from when I was at school, Dad would go round with his little pot of Polyfiller, filling in the cracks and rubbing them down. Of course, he never had time to actually decorate, because, didn't he 'have it all on his plate'? Now he had the time. I can remember that he shook with nerves, in anticipation of what he had to do. I helped Dad as best I could at the weekend, but I could only do what he would allow me, which wasn't much, washing down the woodwork, or holding things.

It was painfully slow. Dad would put one sheet of wallpaper up a day. Each piece was measured and re-measured, then checked again, while he read a book on how to do it. Each piece of wallpaper was put up as perfectly as was humanly possible. He was a bundle of nerves the whole time, which was reflected in his mood before starting. He would put off starting each day for as long as possible, doing unnecessary tasks, like writing and re-writing a shopping list, until Mum would have enough and tell him to get on with it. Of course, that was like lighting the blue touch paper and standing back.

This was a daily occurrence. The rows were frequent, and his moods always foul. He would criticise everyone else for the slightest imperfection of what ever they were doing, because it was easier to pass judgement on everyone else's limitations, than to admit to his own. Eventually the lounge was finally completed. It took most of the eighteen months that Dad was unemployed, but the finished product was as good as, if not better, than one would get from a professional. The fact that it took so much out of him to do, having to cope with his anxiety and perfectionism, coupled with his obsessive, compulsive personality disorder, made it an even more admirable accomplishment.

After eighteen months of getting nowhere with job applications, Mum advised Dad to go shop to shop to see if there were any manual labour jobs. I think they had both come to the same conclusion that Dad wasn't going to get a clerks position. He had never done manual labour, and was really the wrong age to start, but this was probably his only option.

After trying most of the shops in St. Albans, he ventured into Boots, and spoke to the manager. As luck would have it, there was a vacancy. It involved unloading cages of goods from lorries and pushing these into the store for the shelf fillers. The job also included sweeping and cleaning and he would be responsible for locking up at night. It was hard, backbreaking work but when asked, Dad said he was fit enough to do it. I think the manager felt sorry for him, as he knew how hard it was to get a job at that time of life, so he took him on. Dad was very grateful for the job, but he found it very physically demanding. He had to start around 7.30 in the morning and work until about 6 o'clock at night. The early starts were very hard for Dad. Like me, Dad was not a morning person.

After he had finished his work for the day and locked up, he had to get whatever shopping was needed. He was getting home about 7 o'clock at night exhausted. This proved to be a problem on Saturday nights. Saturday night was church night, which started around 7pm. Dad would come home, not have time for his tea, and have to race, (for him!) to try to get Mum and himself to church on time. They were always late. By the time they arrived, the congregation was already sitting down and the sermon had begun. In the Catholic Church, if you hadn't heard the gospel, which comes before the sermon, then you haven't heard the Mass. Mum was all for creeping in and sitting at the back, so that they would not be noticed. Not Dad! He insisted on going right up the front, in order to try to do justice to the Mass. He would be frantically beckoning to Mum to follow him, and getting angry if she pretended not to see him. Therefore, to avoid any further public humiliation, she had to do what he wanted.

The same thing happened if Julie and I were there, which we tried not to be. We went to church at a different time, if we could. To make matters worse, Dad wore shoes with metal heel protectors, so his procession to the front of the church sounded like someone had brought in a horse. So you can imagine, there's the poor old priest, giving his sermon, being drowned out by Dad, clip clopping his way to the front, saying, 'Excuse me, sorry, pardon me', to the parishioners that he was squeezing by, so that he could reach his pew. Mum, meanwhile, was wishing that a hole would open up that she could disappear into.

At the end of the service, Dad would try to make up for the prayers that he missed from the beginning of the Mass and would stay until he had finished. This would go on for ages, with the priests putting their coats on and turning off the lights, hoping he would take the hint. Mum, meanwhile, would get more and more embarrassed, and finally told him that she would wait in the car. This would annoy Dad, so he wouldn't give her the car keys, as a punishment for her harassing him before he was ready. Poor old Mum then had to wait in the freezing cold for 20 or 30 minutes until Dad was good and ready.

On the way home, Dad would insist on filling up with petrol. Saturday nights were very busy at the petrol station we used. The queue of cars stretched out onto the road. After Dad had filled in his form, did his adding up and taking away, the queue was round the block. The hand gestures and language of the other motorists were even more explicit on those nights.

Why, you may ask, didn't they go to church on a Sunday, when Dad didn't have to go to work? Good question. The reason was, after a long and tiring week at work, Dad slept for most of Sunday. He would get up late Sunday morning, have a wash and a shave, and then he would have about an hour before it was lunchtime. He might use this time checking and re-checking bills or bank statements.

After lunch, he would sleep until around 5 o'clock, when he would perhaps work in the garden or 'service' the car. Julie or I would have to hold the torch for him while this was going on, as it would start getting dark before he finished. I have to explain here that Dad called it servicing the car. He didn't do anything mechanical, just the regular maintenance of checking the oil, water and battery fluid. It would take him about an hour to do this, due to Dad's O.C.D. Everything had to be checked and rechecked, which was very boring for the torch holder.

Sunday nights were also bath nights for Dad. However, it was always quite late before he got going. He would have his tea, watch the news, and potter about a bit, before making it to the bathroom. Therefore, it was so late by the time he finished, often midnight, that he didn't have time to clean the bath out after him. So he reasoned that if he left the water in until the next day, that would prevent a tidemark. The next day, after the water had time to stagnate over night, was bath cleaning out day, and I remember Mum, Dad and Julie would take turns doing this. I didn't. You have to draw the line somewhere.

Dad wasn't earning very much money working for Boots, and the job was taking its toll physically, therefore he continued looking through the local papers to see if he could get a less strenuous position. He eventually came across an advert for a car park attendant for the local council. He applied for this job and got it. There was only one drawback. He would have to drive one of their vans. This was a big problem for Dad, as he was not a very confident driver and only drove locally. In this job, he would have to drive outside St. Albans to get to the various car parks. I did a few dummy runs with Dad in our own car to Harpenden and other places to get him used to driving there. He never really got used to it though, and was always a bundle of nerves before setting off.

Apart from the driving aspect of the job, I think Dad quite liked the work. He certainly used to do it better than the other people working there. All they were interested in was skiving off, so it annoyed them when Dad did the job properly. It probably annoyed the motorists that he booked as well, they would have preferred the skivers, but there you are.

I could take it no longer at the benefit office, so I announced to Mum and Dad that I wanted to leave. Well, there was an almighty row. Dad told me that I couldn't leave, that I had a safe career working for the government and that I would get a good pension when I was sixty. Sixty? At this rate, I would be lucky to live until I was twenty-six. Mum was begging me to stay for peace sake. I would hear that plea so often during my life. I left anyway.

I went to Oakland's College and embarked on a secretarial course. But of course, although the location had changed, I had not. I couldn't take anything in, and did less and less of the course, until eventually, all I did was the basic typing course. I passed this, but I think that was more by luck than judgement.

I left the college with meagre qualifications and started looking through the paper to see if there was anything that I could do. I had to apply for a temp job, because if I went for a permanent position the company would ask for my medical record, which would show that I had been under a psychologist for two and a half years and was on permanent medication. Therefore, I applied for a temporary job at Lloyds Bank, for which I was accepted. Unfortunately, they surprised me by saying that they would need my medical history. I supplied my doctor's name, and two weeks later I got a letter through the post saying that the position was no longer available. No shock there then.

I persevered, and applied for a job at The Abbey National Building Society. They wanted someone with key board skills and who was familiar with a computer screen. I still wasn't very motivated about doing anything, especially working in a back office, but I reasoned that if I had a job on the counter, (as when I was working fresh claims in the Benefit Office), the person sitting opposite me would motivate me. I needed that external stimulus. Unlike Lloyds, The Abbey National didn't check my medical background and took me on. I soon realised that they hadn't done me any favours. I had to work with two horrible, bitchy women; Mrs. Keahane, who was in charge of the cashiers, and another woman called Carol, whose surname escapes me. Mrs. Keahane's daughter, by the way, used to bully my sister Julie at school. Like mother like daughter. These two women found out that I had a psychological illness and suffered from anorexia, and made my life a misery. They thought that anyone with a mental illness was a loony and treated me as such.

Despite the fact that I was very unhappy there, I stayed for sixteen months, under a temporary contract. As with the benefit office, The Abbey sent me on courses, and, as in the Benefit Office, I came back from them as ignorant as before I went. I couldn't cope with anything other than the bare basics of the job, and certainly couldn't take anything new in.

One of my biggest regrets regarding my illness was not getting a driving licence. My dream was to become a teacher, pass my test and drive a snazzy sports car. Alas, it wasn't to be. I started learning after I passed my A levels, using my Norbury money to pay for six lessons. Once again fate was against me, as the man that I got to teach me was all wrong for me. It was the same man that taught Dad, (I don't know how he survived that ordeal), but he had the wrong method of teaching for someone as sensitive as me. He didn't believe in a gentle approach, but instead threw me in at the deep end and was quite blasé about the fact that I said I was terrified. In fact, I used to stop the car by stalling it. He didn't believe I was scared as, because I was tense, my foot pushed the accelerator to the floor, and we used to bomb along the road with all the trees and bushes flying by in a blur; it was like something out of Wacky Races. He thought I was over confident, but nothing could be further from the truth.

One day he took me down St. Peter's street, in St. Albans, which is a busy road at the best of times; that day, though, was market day. There were cars coming from all angles and I was petrified. When we came to a roundabout, I didn't have a clue what to do, so I kept going... straight in front of all the on coming traffic. There was an Express Dairies milk float coming towards me and to avoid turning us into a milk shake, he ended up on the grass bank of the roundabout. Meanwhile we carried on at the speed of light towards all the market stalls. There were shoppers and market stallholders throwing themselves out of the way of our tearaway car. It was like one of those car chase scenes in a Hollywood film. To this day, I don't know how someone wasn't killed and that we didn't end up wrapped around a lamppost. Beginners luck, I suppose. The driving instructor wasn't too impressed though. He thought he was a goner, and had sweat pouring out of every orifice; (at least, I think it was sweat). Bearing in mind he had taught Dad for God knows how long, and therefore he wasn't easy to shake up, I managed to do it. Luckily for him, I was just about to leave for Digby Stuart, so I couldn't have any more lessons. Not that I wanted any more. That experience put me off learning, for a while at least.

I started learning again while I was at Abbey National. I had driving lessons with a different instructor this time, a Mr. Milne, as I think my original instructor had retired to a French penal colony for a quiet life. My sister Julie and I decided to share lessons, as we were both nervous and would bolster each other's confidence. Unfortunately, I did no better this time as I still couldn't take things in, and I used to dread these lessons. I would rather have had all my teeth pulled out. I used to binge before I went and binge when I came home to try to get through them. I persevered for about eighteen months, which was really a waste of my time and certainly a waste of money.

Dad also attempted to teach me, which really was the blind leading the blind. He was bad with his nerves and couldn't cope with driving himself. In fact, he should have his own entry in The Guinness Book of Records for the most attempts at the driving test. He had about ten, and in the end the white-faced examiner said to him, 'Well, I'll pass you Mr. Kennedy, but you must promise me that you'll keep practising before you go far'.

Anyway, Dad couldn't teach me, and we had rows galore, ending with me getting out of the car, slamming the door, and walking home. I never did get my licence, although Julie did. She persevered with Mr. Milne and Dad, and she has now become a local driver herself. If I promised a driving examiner that I would stay local, would he pass me as well?

The Christian social group that I was a member of joined other Catholic groups that came together every Easter for an event called The Easter Gather, which was held in the All Saints Pastoral Centre in St. Albans. This ran from Maundy Thursday until Easter Day, following the Passion, death and resurrection of Christ, with a Mass on the Sunday. On the Saturday evening, there was a party. This was very 'safe', as it was all religion based, supervised by priests, and I was mixing with my type of people.

One of the founder members of contact was a man called Greg Peachey. On this occasion, he had brought his sister Kathy along. I saw this little innocent looking girl standing by herself in the corner, pretending to enjoy herself but wishing she could be anywhere else. I could see myself in her. I went straight over to talk to her, and started a friendship that has lasted to this day. Kathy had even less of a social life than I did. She would stay at home with her mum and dad, except on a Saturday when she would walk round the shops with her sister. She was extremely shy and innocent, and the nicest person you could meet. We hit it off straight away, and found that we had a lot in common, including that we were both learning to drive, and hating it.

Kathy lived in Bedford and was, and still is, very religious and regularly went to church. That was the extent of her social life though. Greg took her on as a kind of project, to get her to come out of her shell and to make some friends. He meant well, but he would take her to things like the Easter Gather, and leave her there to fend for herself. She was too shy to talk to anyone, and so hated it. Greg used to bring her to his flat, also in St. Albans, and invite a load of his male friends along, who were completely frightening to Kathy, and then go out and leave her with them. After a while of seeing that this wasn't working, Greg would ring me up and ask if Kathy could come round our house for the afternoon.

Occasionally she was allowed to come on the train to St. Albans to visit us on her own. Julie and I would meet her at the station, and her father would meet her back at Bedford station. Before she met me, Kathy had never even been on a train. That was the start of Kathy's social life. She has stuck by me thick and thin ever since, and is the best friend anyone could ever have.

Towards the end of my time at The Abbey National, I went on a holiday with Dana, Andy, Ita, Sister Madeline and a few others. We went to a convent in the Lake District, called The Hyning, which used to be Sir Robert Peel's house. There was a guest cottage in the grounds next to the convent, and that's where we stayed. That was a really happy holiday for me and I thoroughly enjoyed it. I used to watch the nuns going about their business in calm tranquillity as I had experienced at Roehampton while I was at Digby, and in my naïveté, I thought that if I joined them my life would be all calm and tranquil.

However, it's a bit like anywhere you go on holiday; with the sun shining, no pressure and having a good time, you think that if you were to live there it would be like that all the time. Unfortunately, life's not like that, at least for me it isn't. When you move somewhere else all your baggage goes with you. You just have to unpack it all the other end. Nevertheless, in my innocent way, I thought it would all get better if I lived with these serene nuns. So I did a deal with God and said that if I gave six months of my life serving these nuns, would He make me better? I thought that quite a good bargain, but obviously, God did not.

I wrote with great anticipation to the nuns in Hyning, who were unaware of my health problems, and offered my services as a Guest Mistress. They were delighted to have me come and work for them. Unfortunately, the guesthouse in Hyning was closed for the month of August in order that the nuns could have their own holiday, so they suggested that I went to their other convent, St. Bernard's in Slough, Berkshire, until it reopened.

I can't say that Mum and Dad were over the moon when I told them of my decision. I think Dad just thought, 'Oh, here we go again, what will she do next?' But really, I think he had just about given up on me. I had failed at everything else I tried to do; this was just one more thing.

I received a letter from St. Bernard's with directions on how to get there, so off I went, once more convinced that this would be my answer. I got off the bus at Langley, walked to the convent, and was most impressed at what I saw. It was a very imposing stately home, in its own grounds. The main house comprised of the Grammar school, the reception area, the nuns community lounge, a guest dining room for visitors, the kitchens, a private drawing room for the nuns, the chapel, then up the sweeping staircase were two guest bedrooms, a washroom and laundry room. Linking this building was another wing, which housed the nuns private sleeping quarters.

Behind the main building were orchards in extensive grounds, and behind those, other fruit and vegetables were also grown. At the back of that was another building, which was a small private prep school, which the nuns also ran. Across the courtyard from the manor house was a separate building, which used to be the stables. The lower floor was used for storing the fruit and vegetables. Above this, (in what used to be the hayloft), there was a guest lounge and three bedrooms. These rooms were for visitors to the nuns, friends and relatives, plus one room at the end, which was Teresa's bed-sitter.

Teresa had worked for the nuns for years, although I don't think she was ever a nun. I got the impression that she didn't have anywhere else to live, so the nuns let her stay in the guesthouse. She was a very dour Scots woman and I didn't like her very much, (I think she felt that I was a threat to her), but I later learnt a lot about the other nuns from her.

Continuing the tour, if you walked out of the convent grounds and along the road, you arrived at another large detached house, also part of the convent, which was where the Japanese students lived. There were ten of these Japanese students that came every year on a bursary, to perfect their English and learn about English life and how to entertain English businessmen and so forth, so that they could go back to Japan and make good marriages. There was also a Japanese teacher that came with them who taught them other subjects in Japanese.

When I arrived, I was given one of the guest rooms in the main building. I recall that it was Bank Holiday that day, and the nuns had half a day off. Two priests from Africa, Father Prosper and Father Boniface and me, were invited to join the nuns for a bit of a get together and a singsong. These two priests were quite high up in the priesthood and were very nice to me. I later found out that when they eventually went back to Zaire they became Bishops.

It all seemed wonderful at first. I did a few odd jobs around the place until it was time for me to go to Hyning. I remember it was apple-picking time, which I helped with. I was enjoying myself and looking forward to when I would be going to the Lake District when all my problems would be over. However, after a couple of nights at Slough I had a very unnerving experience. I was asleep in bed and was woken by the sensation of someone moving about. Someone was trying to get into bed with me. I could feel them moving about on top of me and then getting under the covers. It was terrifying. I couldn't move, couldn't cry out, I was frozen in terror. I was literally paralysed with fear.

Eventually I managed to emit a scream and the person sprung off me and headed for the door. I shouted out, 'Who are you, what do you want?', and in the darkness, a woman's voice answered, 'Oh, don't worry about it, you were dreaming, go back to sleep'. With that, she left. I got a good look at who it was, however, as the light from the corridor lit up her face. It was one of the novices.

The next day it so happened that I was assigned to go with this novice and another nun to clean the chapel. While there, I challenged her about incident of the night before. When I asked her why she tried to get into my bed, the novice and the nun exchanged a meaningful look with each other and the novice denied all knowledge of it, suggesting that I dreamed it all. The nun backed up the novice and said that of course I was dreaming. I knew it happened, that it wasn't a dream, but I also knew by the meaningful glance to each other that the nun knew more than she let on and was obviously protecting the novice. Whether it had happened before in the past, I don't know, but it was vehemently denied that it happened that night. I know what happened, and will never forget that frightening experience.

The time came for me to leave St. Bernard's, so off I set, full of hope and expectation for a renewed life. I arrived at Carnforth station, near Hyning, (where Brief Encounter was filmed) and was met by one of the nuns who brought me back to the guesthouse, which I was going to run. I was given a room in the attic. My job was to look after the guests and do the housework. I expect you can see the flaw in my plan already. I couldn't cope with dusting or hoovering and felt totally overwhelmed with it all. I was left on my own to do everything, the nuns being on one side of a wall, with me the other. This wasn't what I wanted. Where was the peace and serenity that God was going to give me? Far from feeling calm and tranquil, I felt stressed and anxious.

After only a week or two, I went to see the Mother Superior, Sister Philippa, who was a lovely lady. I told her that it wasn't working and that I couldn't cope and that I was very lonely, so she liaised with Sister Mary Edmond, who was the Mother Superior at Slough, and arranged for me to go back there.

When I returned to St. Bernard's, I was given a room in the small guest house in the old stable block, next to Teresa's bed sitter, and a job was created for me. I was to help the woman whose name I don't recall, who was in charge of the Japanese student's house. She was an ex United Reform Minister turned Catholic. My other job was to go to the prep school to help serve the dinners. My food problem at this time was as bad as ever, so the fact that I was allowed into the pantry to help myself to food was not a good idea. It would be akin to letting an alcoholic have the keys to the off licence. I was getting through catering size bowls of custard. I'm sure they were wondering where all the food was going, as the more unhappy I got, the more I ate; I was very unhappy!

The majority of the nuns who I met were very nice to me, but there were others whom I could tell were very unhappy, and were only there because they felt it was their duty. One nun, in fact, told me just that. She said that life in a convent wasn't all that it was cracked up to be, but she had made her decision and now she had to stick to it. The longer one stayed there, the more apparent it became that all was not sweetness and light for some of them. I got some hostility from these unhappy women, especially one French nun, who worked in the kitchens. She was always bitchy to me and asked me if I wanted to be a nun. When I told her that, no I didn't, she said, 'Well why are you here then? You should be out in the community, getting married and having children. You shouldn't be here'. I felt that she was implying that I shouldn't be there sponging off them.

One of the nicest nuns I got to know was Sister Mary. Whereas all the other nuns wore their habits, Sister Mary did not. I later learned from Teresa that she had had a breakdown and couldn't cope with the rigors of being a nun. However, to compensate for this, she would work harder than all the others from morning to night, doing all the jobs no one else wanted to do. In my opinion, she was the most saintly of all the nuns. Teresa told me that on rare occasions she did wear the habit, but that was when her illness got particularly bad.

Once or twice a day, the nuns would feed the down and outs of the area. They would come to the main entrance and be given food. One day one of them got into the guest block, where I lived, as it was quite easy to do. Whoever it was had gone into one of the toilets and smeared all the walls, the floors and even the ceiling with excrement. The stench was overpowering, and it was a disgusting sight. Teresa came and got me to clean it off. I told her that I couldn't do it, and wouldn't do it even if it meant that I had to leave the convent. Well, along came Sister Mary who did it without a murmur. She really was a living saint.

Many of the nuns were quite mannish. Two in particular used to follow each other around wherever they went. They were forever stroking each other and going off together with their arms linked. There was no doubt that these two loved each other, although how far that 'love' went, I don't know. I was quite shocked at this behaviour though, as it was against convent rules to get attached to anyone. They were supposed to devote their love to God.

There were also two little twins, who were in their seventies, who would follow each other around and not let the other out of their sight. They never spoke to anyone while I was there and I got the impression that they had become nuns after getting a convent education because they couldn't cope with life on the outside.

Meanwhile, I was very lonely, the depression was black, and I was on tablets that were having a horrendous effect on me and not really helping. I could see no escape from my mental torment. I remember one awful Christmas I spent there. I had built up a bit of a rapport with the ex United Reform Minister who ran the guesthouse, and she wanted me to help with the Christmas dinner at the Japanese house and to look after the students in the evening. I think that she wanted to go out with a priest friend of hers. I got the impression that she wanted something to come of their relationship, but I knew that it would never happen. Unfortunately, I was very ill Christmas Eve and in a pit of depression walked into Slough to the Catholic Church to make a thorough confession, vowing to make a new start. I knew that Gluttony was a sin and felt that if I confessed my sins I would be helped. However, when I arrived back home at the convent my mind was in such torment, even more so than before I left, that I had a massive binge to try and quell my tortured mind.

I would like to explain a bit about binge eating. Most people, I'm sure, would not really understand. It's not just eating a Mars Bar when you're fed up, or feeling guilty if you have a cream cake. It's eating until you can't eat anymore, and then eating some more. Food is stuffed down to try and suppress whatever anguish is going through your mind at the time, in the vain attempt to make yourself happy. Imagine how you feel after a big Christmas dinner. You feel full, but nevertheless, you have a pudding after, then later on maybe some nuts and chocolates. You feel fit to bursting, don't you? Multiply that three times, and you might get some idea how I felt. You lie down, being unable to stand, and your stomach swells up. A nauseating smell emits from every pore. You are unable to move, and then you black out.

The best way to explain it is to compare it with drinking. An alcoholic is a binge drinker. If someone drinks too much, they pass out and wake up feeling rough the next day. It is exactly like that with binge eating. I have slept for 48 hours after a binge. Then when you wake up you feel sick, bloated and unable to eat anything for days. That is why I am not 28 stone now, that and the fact that I massively abused laxatives.

That is what happened to me that Christmas Eve. I passed out at 4pm in the evening and woke up at 5pm on Christmas Day. I hastily made my way to the Japanese house, but turned up just in time for dinner to be over. I was obviously too late to be any help, but the ex united reform woman knew I was sick, and was very understanding when I told her what had happened. She encouraged me to go to church as she said that I couldn't miss Mass on Christmas day. I arrived at the church late and stood at the back for the last part of the Mass. I was very religious back then, and therefore felt that I had hit rock bottom by not being able to get to Mass on Christmas day. That was one of the worst Christmases I had ever had, and one that I will never forget. However, it was not the worst; that would come later.

Just before Christmas, the Reverend Mother told me that I would have to move out of my room in the convent in the New Year, as they needed the room. She offered me a job as an assistant in the prep school and had sent out letters to all the parents to the effect that there would be a new teacher in the New Year; however, she said that I would have to find alternative accommodation. She said that she had spoken to Teresa and had found out that there was a woman she knew in the parish that had a room to let. So I went along to see this person, who lived in Langley, about three miles from the convent.

The woman was quite elderly and somewhat disabled. She told me that she wanted not so much a lodger, as a companion, which I felt unhappy about. It meant that I would be at the school all day and have to spend my evenings with her watching the television. She told me that one of the reasons she wanted a companion was that she was frightened of being on her own, due to her violent son-in-law. It transpired that her daughter had broken up with him and she came periodically to stay with her mum. The old lady had, naturally, taken her daughter's side, and so the son-in-law had it in for the old lady, as well as the daughter. He tried on several occasions to make her life a misery. He would break in, in the middle of the night, and wreck the place. She told me she had to have locks replaced and windows repaired where he had broken them.

While she was pointing out various parts of the house that he had smashed up, she told me not to worry about it. She said that it wouldn't be me that he would vent his anger on, but her. She said that it was very noisy and very frightening while it was going on, but I wasn't to be concerned about it. Well, that was a great relief, I'm sure. I was over the moon that while the place was being smashed up all around me by a maniac, I could still sit and carry on watching Coronation Street, twiddling my thumbs, because I was told he wasn't angry at me.

If that wasn't bad enough, she also told me that because she didn't use much milk, there would be a system where she would mark off on the bottle what she used, and I would mark off what I used, then I would pay the difference. That would apply to everything I had there. None of this really made me want to be this woman's companion. Because of my illness I wasn't very good company at the best of times. The fact that I would have to sit there night after night, marking the food and drink that I had, totting up how much I owed her, while waiting for the glass to smash, indicating that the loony son in law was back, was not exactly a prospect that I looked forward to with bliss. Suffice to say, I didn't stay with her.

There was a little Japanese teacher called Miyuki who had come to work at the school. She reminded me a lot of my friend Kathy. I befriended her and rashly, I invited her to spend New Year at our house in St. Albans. I did it to rekindle my now defunct social life. One thing I can tell you about my family, you don't spring surprises on them like that. I could tell they were none too pleased when I turned up with my new friend, although to their credit, they were very nice to her and never let their displeasure show.
That's not to say there wasn't a fair amount of arguments and discussions about what I was doing and what I was going to do. Mum and Dad were at their wits end worrying about the mess my life was in and how it was going to be resolved. I can remember New Year's Eve, with Mum, Dad and I in the lounge having a heart to heart, while we left Miyuki on her own in the dining room watching T.V.

When we joined her later, to our horror, there was a sex film showing. My little Japanese friend was sitting, goggle eyed, at a pair of buttocks wobbling about on the T.V with a lot of moaning and gasping going on. I don't know if she thought that was how we celebrated New Year in England, but she was nice enough not to say anything.

Miyuki stayed with us for a couple of days, much to Mum and Dad's consternation, and we all had to put on a brave face and smile like all was well. Of course, all was not well, and I was in a dreadful state. I couldn't go back, I was far too ill. What were we going to do? My friend Dana came to the rescue. She took Dad and I, along with Miyuki, back to Slough in her car. I don't know what Miyuki thought about her New Year with these mad English people, but I'm sure she entertained her family with it once she got home.

I tried to explain to the Reverend Mother that I wasn't well, that the tablets that I was on were having a devastating effect on me; that I couldn't cope with life there, and that I was sorry, but I wouldn't be taking up her offer as an assistant. She took it in good faith, although I'm not sure if she really understood. Once again, I came home with my tail between my legs. A failure yet again.

LEAVING HOME

'Well, what are you going to do with your life then?' asked Dad. Good question. Everything I had tried to do since leaving school had ended in failure. My ongoing problems: the depression, the fatigue, my problems around food, coupled with the fact that I didn't function at all in the mornings, meant that I was more or less unemployable. I just couldn't cope with ordinary life. I was backwards and forwards to the G P, who really just tried one drug after another on me, none of which worked. However, I am not one to just curl up and die. I would do something, although I didn't know what.

I ventured down to Blue Arrow, a recruiting agency in St. Albans, to see what they had to offer. I didn't really have much in the way of qualifications for the jobs they had on offer. They put me on their books, but I didn't really hold out much hope. What could I do? I could barely hold myself together, living day to day. They told me of another recruitment agency in Fleetville that I could try while they were waiting to fix me up with a suitable position.

I went to this agency, which was situated in the drabbest building in the seediest part of St. Albans. You had to wipe your feet when you came out. This agency recruited for industrial temps. These were jobs that were only really filled by illegal immigrants, ex convicts and the like. How low had I sunk? However, I was desperate to be employed at something and to be able to pay my way, just to get back a little self worth.

As I was unable to do anything before midday, I would arrive in the afternoon and wait around until there was a job. I couldn't really speak to anyone there, as I seem to remember being the only person with English as a first, or even second, language. The jobs would run from about four in the afternoon until ten at night. Bear in mind that we weren't paid for waiting around, or even while travelling to the various factories. We only were paid while we were actually at work, and even then not much. We also had very little break times while at these factories. You had to make up your mind whether to spend your ten minutes having a cup of tea or to go to the toilet.

They told me I was being emergency taxed, plus they would take out my national insurance. I later found out they kept my tax and insurance. At the end of a hard week, I was lucky to clear £40. (They have since been closed down, due to illegal business practices, thank God).

We would all go in a minibus, which had no tax or insurance, was full of rust and holes, and was driven by a man with an alcohol problem who didn't actually have a licence. He was nearly always the worst for wear. The company didn't seem to worry about trifling things like that. I'm fortunate to have survived the journeys. I did various jobs for these people, which usually ran for a week at a time. Once I worked in an apple factory, packing apples into cartons, with reminiscences of my time holding apples for Dad. That was where the similarity ended, however. I wouldn't have lasted long if I had to measure each apple with a ruler and setsquare before carefully placing each one an inch apart. Everything was rush, rush, rush.

I also worked at a cheese factory, packing cheese. If any of the cheese fell on the floor, we were not allowed to put it in the bin. Instead, it would be grated up and sold as grated cheese

I did get a few jobs through Blue Arrow. I was registered with them on the industrial side as well as clerical. One of the industrial jobs I got was in the kitchens at St. Albans city hospital. This was very hard manual labour. If I were an all in wrestler I might have coped, but I was a seven and a half stone weakling, with numerous psychological problems. This job nearly killed me. I had to hump great huge sacks of cabbages, then cut them and prepare them for the meals.

Anyone who has visited a hospital will know of the all-pervading smell of antiseptic and boiled cabbage. I was responsible for the latter. I was also responsible for making the toast. You can imagine how much toast I had to make. The grill was so large, that with my arms stretched to their fullest extent, I could just reach either end of it. You could fit two loaves of sliced bread at a time into it. The heat emitting from this thing was so fierce, you actually ended up with a grilled face.

I was also in the serving up assault course. Have you ever watched Candid Camera, where a temp is put on a conveyor belt and told to put the cream on the cakes as they go past, only for the line to go faster and faster until all the cakes fall off the end? Well, it wasn't much different here. The supervisor would stand at the top, and shout out each person's dinner. As that plate came past you, you had to put that ingredient on to the plate. The trouble was, she was at the top of the conveyor belt, calling out all these meals, but by the time the plate got to you, she was about six dinners in front. You had to have a really good memory to know what ingredient went on what plate. Each person on the conveyor belt was responsible for three or four ingredients, one or two ingredients for the dinner, and one or two ingredients for the pudding, which you had in front of you in huge vats. Therefore, you might be in charge of liver, the ubiquitous cabbage, gravy and custard. Also, bear in mind that the majority of people working there were from ethnic minorities and could hardly speak English. You're way ahead of me here, aren't you? If you were not on top of it all, it would be quite easy to give someone liver and custard, or apple pie and gravy; or if they were very unlucky, both.

I also did the washing up. I was in charge of the pots, which all had to be done by hand, using scouring pads. There were dozens of these to do. There was no mechanical help; the dishwashers were only for cups and plates. I worked from seven thirty in the morning until five in the evening, and by the end of the week I was completely shattered. I would have to sleep for most of the weekend to recover. I did three separate weeks altogether in the hospital kitchens. I really do admire people who do this job day in and day out. They're soul-destroying jobs with very little money. I did various menial jobs with the agency, each as bad as the other.

Meanwhile, I was determined that I would have to make a new start in a place of my own. I knew that Dad was coming up to retirement soon, and in all honesty, I don't think that I could have faced life at home with him there full time. One of the Westminster Missionaries had a flat in a place called Martins Court, in St. Albans. I asked him how he got it and he told me he just put his name down with the letting agent and suggested I did the same, which I did. I heard nothing and forgot all about it. But now that Dad's retirement was imminent I decided to go to the manager in charge of letting to see how things stood.

When I phoned, I found out that there was a different man in charge. His name was Rasheed and it sounded like he was in a terrible mess. He couldn't find my file, or anybody's file, come to that. He asked me when I put my name on the waiting list and I told him two years earlier. This was true, but you are supposed to renew it yearly, which I hadn't done. However, because he couldn't find my file he wasn't to know that.

'Well, if you've been on the waiting list two years, you should have been given a place by now,' he said. I didn't argue.

Now, there was a procedure at Martins Court, wherein the first place you're given is a shared flat. After sharing for about five years you can then move on to a studio flat. Then, after an eternity, if you're lucky, you can move into a two floor flat for one. These were like gold dust at Martins Court, as there were only about half a dozen of them.

'It just so happens,' said Rasheed, 'that there is a vacancy in one of the shared flats. If you come along, I will show it to you'. I agreed to go, but I was very apprehensive. I never had much luck sharing in the past and didn't hold out much hope here.

Martins Court is quite large and imposing, and inside it is a warren of dark, meandering passages. Ideal drug dealers' territory, which indeed I later found out was exactly what it was. I was taken to this flat and introduced to the occupants. There was one man, who had elected himself as chairman and representative for the group, and a girl called Linda. There was also another girl, but she was out at the time. The situation was quite bizarre and reminded me of the woman who wanted a companion in Slough. The 'Chairman' of the group informed me that the phone bill was in his name. So if I wanted to make a call, he would stand next to me with a stopwatch and time each call I made. He would then charge me accordingly. I asked him what would happen if we wanted to make a call while he wasn't there. He said we couldn't. I have a feeling that he would do very well out of this deal. He would probably get most of his own calls free, with us mugs paying his bit. He was also in charge of the water bill. He wanted me to ration the water and tell him when I was going to have a bath and how much water I was going to use. I don't know how he was going to see if I was telling the truth. Come in with a ruler, no doubt.

If all that seems far-fetched, the best bit is that he said he owned the sofa. He said that if I wanted to sit on it he would charge me rent. He had it all worked out, so much per hour charged weekly. I didn't tell him what I thought.

When I went back to Rasheed, he was beaming all over his face.

'Good news', he said, 'I've just heard from the tenants of the flat you just visited, and they said that you're exactly the right person they want to share with them'.

'Well, they might think I'm suitable for them,' I said, 'but they're not suitable for me. There's no way am I going to share in that flat.'

He was taken aback at this. 'Well what do you want then'? He asked.

'I want a place of my own', I said. To say he was stunned at this would be an understatement.

Single flats were very scarce, but as luck would have it, there was one vacant at that moment. Rasheed asked me if I would like to view it. I think the smile I gave him was a good enough answer. As you can imagine, it was unprecedented to offer an outsider one of these large flats. People who have been sharing for years with the likes of 'The Chairman' would sell their grannies for them. I think he broke the rules because he secretly fancied me. Later on, he tried to get friendly with me, and made any excuse to come up to my flat. He used to tell me that I had lovely eyes, and asked if I was related to The Kennedy's, (as if I could be related to one of the richest families in America and live in a housing association flat.) I didn't fancy him. I was always nice to him, but I didn't want any sort of relationship with him. He eventually got the picture and gave up on me.

I went to look round the flat with Dad. He was very wary of me living on my own, and thought that I would be better off at home where I could be looked after. Also he couldn't understand why I would want to pay rent out of my meagre part time work, when I could live for free at home. I knew all this to be true, and tell the truth, I was in two minds about going. I was very scared about going it alone, but I knew that I had to try. I knew that I'd had two abortive attempts at leaving home, once at Digby and once with the nuns; but I also knew that if I didn't go now I never would, and would spend the rest of my life at home and unhappy.

Dad and I would have been at each other's throat once he had retired and we were under each other's feet all day. I don't think he would accept that fact, and never really understood my decision. Anyhow, we went to view this flat one evening. It was quite dark when we got there and there were no light bulbs in the place, so we couldn't see a thing. We were feeling our way round it like Braille. Based on it feeling all right, I took the flat. However, on seeing it in daylight, it didn't look so good. It was a very dark flat, having only one small window high up on one wall, which overlooked a number of trees. Even on a sunny day, it took on the appearance of midwinter. The paintwork was also very drab but my two friends, Dana and Andy, volunteered to come round to help me decorate it.

I'm afraid I wasn't being very fair to these two as I was too ill and tired to help them. I think this peeved them a bit. After all, they were both in full time work and gave all their spare time up to help decorate my flat, but I was never there. They eventually finished the hallway, the living area, the staircase and upper landing. Although they never said anything, I could see they were annoyed that I never helped them and I can understand that. But there was nothing I could do. That was, and is, the nature of my illness. I'm always willing to help and put in my 100%, but sometimes I'm just not able to.

After I moved in, Uncle Bert and Dad did the remaining painting. Bert painted my bathroom, kitchen and bedroom, and Dad glossed all the remaining doors. I know this was hard for my dad to do, but he, like everyone else, was doing it for me. I can't thank them all enough.

Before I moved in, Dad was busy getting to know one of the neighbours. Or at least they were getting to know him. Let me explain. One day, while I was at work, Dad went round to my flat to check out the central heating or the water or something. He wandered upstairs into the bedroom that had a door leading on to a patio. This patio was shared with the next-door neighbour, whose bedroom door also led onto it. Dad strolled out onto the patio to see my next-door neighbour, Jackie, sunbathing. Dad didn't bat an eyelid, and asked Jackie about the stopcock or whatever. She told him what she knew and he went back inside.

Jackie, being quite a shy person, decided that it was time to call it a day on her sunbathing, so she got up and went in to her flat to get out of her bathing suit and get dressed. Well, Dad had a follow up question, (he always did), and went back out onto the patio. He saw that Jackie had gone into her flat, so followed her into her bedroom. This poor girl was now stark naked. She saw Dad coming in and promptly wrapped herself in her curtains. This wasn't going to put Dad off, though. He just carried on with his query about water meters and stopcocks, with poor old Jackie wrapped in her curtains, trying to answer his questions. I bet she wondered what sort of a person was going to be moving in next door. Only Dad could get away with being in a young, naked, girls bedroom and talk about stopcocks. I don't think Mum was too impressed when she found out though.

So there I was, in my own little flat, ready to start a new life. Julie stayed with me for the first weekend to help me unpack and settle in, but after that, I was on my own. After the first night, I realised how much I was missing Mum, as I have always been very close to her. I came down in the morning to find the coffee cup I had used the night before, still on the sink not washed up. It hit home then just what Mum did for me, and that I now had to cope alone. Could I though, that was the question. I wasn't missing Mum for the washing up she did; in fact I used to help a lot with the housework when I was well enough, it was the whole support system that was now gone. Yes, there were wind-ups and irritations with Dad, (and I couldn't cope with those any more), but now there was just silence.

My flat, as fate would have it, was directly opposite the flat I first viewed, with the 'Chairman' et al. As soon as I moved in, Linda, one of the flatmates, gave me the cold shoulder. I could understand her being miffed with me. After all, she had lived in a shared accommodation for years without being given the chance of a flat of her own, and in I come straight off the street into one of the goldmines. For the first time in my life, I was ahead of the game. That didn't help my encounters with Linda very much though.

Because Martins Court was a warren of corridors, it brought back painful recollections of my schooldays; memories of walking through the hallways, waiting to see if there was anyone round a corner to pick on me. Because of my experiences at school, it didn't take much to trigger the fear again. Although Linda never bullied me as such, she told all her other friends in Martins Court what had happened, and they would give me hurtful looks as well. Once more, through no fault of my own, I was the reject. I was so frightened walking down the corridors to the launderette to do my washing that I eventually gave up and Mum started doing it for me. Dad also used to do his bit by doing all my fruit and veg shopping, and I know this was an extra strain for him. After a hard day on the car parks, he would do all his market shopping, and then all mine. He would go home, barely have time for his tea, before bringing all my shopping to me about 9 o'clock at night. Everyone was doing his or her best to help me cope. My family and friends have done a lot for me over the years, and I can't thank them enough.

COLOURFUL CHARACTERS AND FRIDAY FOLK

Opposite Martins Court was Cell Barnes hospital. This was a hospital for the mentally handicapped. Cell Barnes was more like a village than a hospital, where people with various mental handicaps lived and felt safe. Like in any village, there was a place of worship, and Cell Barnes had a Mass centre. The services were put on primarily for the inpatients of the hospital, although outsiders used to come in to help. Julie and I got to hear of this place and decided that we would go there each Sunday, as no-one knew us or asked any embarrassing questions. The handicapped just accepted you as you were.

The priest, Father George Ennis, was a rather dour and austere person. In a way, his demeanour just made the proceedings funny, because he would go on with the Mass whenever bizarre things happened. Bizarre things always happened.

There were a number of colourful characters from the hospital who would attend these Masses. One of the main personalities was someone whose nickname was Ginger. He used to like dressing up and I think he quite fancied himself as a priest. Obviously, he couldn't take the part of the priest. That job had already gone to someone else, so he took the next best thing, that of altar server. He liked this job, as it involved getting dressed up in the regalia, which was similar to what the priest was wearing.

It was also his job to take the collection. He didn't know a lot about money, but he was better at getting it out of people than Bob Geldof. He would look at what people had put on the collection plate, and if he thought they hadn't put enough in he would say in a loud voice, 'Cor, you're tight aren't you. Go on put some more in. Look how much he's put in Father, he's tight inee'?

Quite often during the Mass, if Ginger got bored, he would turn all the lights out, start stacking the chairs and put away all the altar paraphernalia. Father Ennis carried on regardless, stern face not cracking an inch. When it came to the sermon, Ginger had certain bits he liked. He would proceed in encouraging the priest by shouting out, 'Go on Father, tell 'em the one about the loaves and fishes. Tell 'em about that trick', or, 'Tell 'em about the trick of turning water into wine, that's a goodun'. Sometimes he would say, 'Tell 'em about that woman, you know, that prostitute woman. They'll like that one'.

During all this heckling the priest would carry on as if nothing was happening. Because he was so straight faced and dour, it just made the whole thing even funnier. Trying not to laugh when you're not supposed to makes you want to even more.

There was also a little leering man called George, although he was better known as 'Hans Roaming'. This was because he would take every opportunity to grope the women whenever he could. Instead of saying hello and shaking hands, he would grope your bust. You had to be fast when he approached, and take hold of his hands, before he got a couple of handfuls. The middle of the service was George's favourite bit. That is when everyone turns to everyone else to say, 'Peace be with you', and shakes his or her hand. Well, this was just an open invitation for old George. To him, all the women were saying, 'Peace be with you, and do you want a piece?' You had to be right on your guard with him. Anyone new to the Mass centre was in for a shock if she didn't know what to expect.

There was a woman, a gypsy called Rene, who had a stock phrase, which you had to respond to properly. The phrase was, 'Who touches the organ'? Now there wasn't an organ to touch, but nevertheless, you had to answer, 'The organist touches the organ'. Any other reply, such as 'We haven't got an organ', or 'Someone else touches the organ', or 'Go and ask George', would make this lady very distressed. She would keep on asking, 'Who touches the organ?' until you gave her the correct response. She would then wander off quite happily, to confront someone else with the same question.

Rene was also the flower supplier. Not officially, you understand. She had it in her head that you couldn't have a Mass without flowers. So she would make sure there were flowers, by nicking them out of the hospital garden. She would then proceed up to the altar, halfway through Mass, to shove this illicit bunch of daffodils under the nose of the priest. 'Here you are then Father, here's yer flowers'. Poor old Father Ennis then had to try and find somewhere for these flowers, as there were no vases.

'Thank you Rene', he would say.

'That's all right Father,' she would say, 'who touches the organ?'

There was another great character called Andrew Unsworth, who would time his arrival to perfection, to coincide with the collection plate going round. Not that he was keen on donating, far from it. He would wait until it was his turn for the collection plate, so that he could take money out. He thought this was a very good deal. He could get all he wanted to use in the tuck shop.

So imagine the scene. There was Ginger taking the collection, (if he hadn't turned off all the lights and packed everything up by then), berating the parishioners for being tight, and meanwhile Andrew was helping himself to his sweet money. If the priest saw Andrew come in, he would order him out. Nine times out of ten though, Andrew would ignore this and carry on with his own charity work. However, if he was thwarted with his enterprising scheme, he would wait until the end of the service, (which may or may not be a long wait, depending on how bored Ginger was), to accost the parishioners on the way out with, 'Cup of tea, cup of tea', with his hand outstretched. I'm sure he is quite rich by now.

There was a woman called Kitty, who would speak about herself in the third person. 'Kitty went to the shops yesterday' or 'Kitty had a nice dinner last night'. Kitty also suffered greatly from flatulence. Most people tried to avoid sitting next to her. Quite often though, she would come and sit next to me. I would be sitting there trying to listen to the Mass, knowing what was going to come next. She would let one or two squeaks out, like someone letting the air out of a balloon, then suddenly let out a resounding fart accompanied with the inevitable pong, turn to the person next to her, (usually me), and say in a loud voice, 'Do you want to go to the toilet now?' I hope the rest of the congregation didn't think the niff was any of my doing.

There was a couple that went who were obviously very much in love with each other, and would demonstrate this fact whenever they could. For example, when the congregation stood up to sing a hymn, this couple would take the opportunity to use the now vacant pew to get on top of each other. I can't listen to 'Mine eyes have seen the glory' without thinking of those two. During prayers, when the congregation had to give their responses, the man had a very endearing habit of waiting until the precise moment before putting his hand up the woman's dress in order to elicit a high-pitched 'Whoop' from her. If he timed it right, she would whoop just as everyone else 'hallelujahed'. The couple's affections carried on even while everyone was queuing up for Holy Communion. They would rummage each other while everyone else pretended they couldn't see them.

On the occasions that Kathy came to stay with me, she would also join Julie and me for Mass. However, as she had led a very sheltered life, we had to prime her before we got to the

Mass centre. We certainly had to keep her away from Hans Roaming. When we took her, her eyes would be like organ stops. She had never seen the like before. She said that she understood, and that these people had their problems, but really it was all beyond her. She still laughs about it now, in between mouthfuls of tranquillisers.

'Friday Folk' was a barn-dancing group that was held every Friday in a church hall in Fleetville, St. Albans. I think it was Mum that told Julie and me about it, as she realised that we needed a social outlet. We were both very nervous about going, especially me with all the bad experiences I had with social events in the past. All the same, I made myself go to try to get myself a life. Julie felt the same way. Dad said that he would take us and bring us back until Julie got a little car of her own.

Everyone there made us very welcome, although most of them were quite different to Julie and I. For a start, they all seemed to have good, well-paid jobs. Having said that, they were all as tight as a drum. They all seemed to have nice cars and big houses, but I remember they were all mortgaged up to the hilt and never put their hands in their pockets to buy a drink. The weekly fee for the club was £2, which included a glass of orange juice. This was just as well, as otherwise they would have all died of thirst.

There were as many eccentric characters here as there were at the Mass centre, but this lot were just a bit richer. My sister and I used to have a bit of fun by giving people names to go with their characteristics. One couple we named 'Mannish Woman' and 'Gypsy man'. They were both quite bohemian. She was very hairy and a bit dirty and had no dress sense. She would wear Moses sandals with big woolly jumpers and floral skirts.

She was living with Gypsy man, who was just as dirty and even hairier. Even though they had a lot of money, they bought all their clothes in charity shops. It seems they didn't sell soap in the charity shops they frequented.

There was a little, round, man, with a little round apple face, called Richard. He was Indian and quite pompous. He was chief engineer at a big company. I found out later that he also fancied me.

There was an old fashioned, rather precise, lady called Anne. She was very nice, but also very tight. She was a librarian and quite well off, but she would wear the same dress week in week out, that she had made herself.

Stuart was tall and thin and a bundle of nerves. Although he had a good job, he was probably the least well off of any of them. He was also a terrible bore. If he told you a story, you would have to force yourself to stay awake. He was also terribly precise. If you made an off the cuff remark to him, for example, 'It's freezing out today', he would say, 'Oh, I wouldn't say it was freezing. I haven't actually seen any water on the road frozen. I would say it's about 2 degrees'. Stuart also fancied his chances with me, but more about that later.

Most of the people I met at Friday Folk wore the same clothes every week. Some of them may have even washed them first. Harold was no exception. He was a college lecturer, and in all the time I knew him, he wore the same pair of brilliant bright green trousers. I can't remember what he taught at college, (perhaps it was penny pinching) but I'm sure that if he wore the same clothes there, most of the students would be concentrating on his garb rather than what he was saying.

Many of the members who came week in week out couldn't dance to save their lives. You would watch them and wonder what music they were listening to, as the beat certainly had nothing to do with the movements they were making. David Brent dancing in 'The Office' was like Fred Astaire compared to them. The sad part was they all thought they were fantastic.

One of these was an Asian man called Abdu. He was a great big bear of a man who had two huge left feet and arms that would wave dangerously near your face. He would clump about during these dances, and it was all you could do to stop yourself ending up black and blue afterwards.

I have been kicked, pummelled, and trodden on so many times, that if people were to see me afterwards they would have thought that I had just come from a self-defence class rather than a dance.

On one occasion, my friend Dana came to a Friday Folk dance. Fresh meat for Abdu. He honed in on poor Dana, who didn't really like dancing but came because I asked her to. He kicked and bashed Dana at every opportunity. At the end of the evening, the barn dance would end in a Polka. A man called Brian and I used to dance this Polka, as we were quite good at it. Poor old Abdu watched us do this and decided that Dana was the perfect partner to show off his skills. The Polka is quite a fast dance, and it takes a lot of co-ordination to do it right. Abdu couldn't co-ordinate walking in a straight line. He grabbed hold of Dana and made off at full tilt across the room. It was like watching a runaway train. They both ended up sprawled on the floor with arms and legs everywhere. It looked more like all in wrestling. After being used as a human battering ram, Dana came off the floor absolutely furious. 'Never again,' she said, 'Never will I be humiliated like that again.'

Another man that was quite a character was someone we named 'Come Hither'. He was a little, quite pompous man, not much personality, but with a very good job. He was probably a banker. I don't know what his real name was, but we named him Come Hither after his mannerisms. If you were doing a dance with him that involved going apart backwards before moving forward again he would beckon you towards him by crooking his finger. He would conduct the whole dance with his finger. Sometimes I felt like conducting it back with two fingers.

There was another man who was very sparse. He was really a man in a boy's body. One night he came with his new girlfriend. Well, this girl was enormous. She was as big as he was little. She could have picked this man up with one arm. The dress she wore could have held its own barn dance. Suffice to say, we named them 'Little and Large'.

Occasionally the church hall that we used for the dances was not available to us. On these occasions we would go round to Anne's house for a get together, as she lived the nearest. Anne was the librarian that wore her own homemade dress, week in week out. She had a very nice house as she was quite well off, but there was a good reason for that. She was as tight as a botox smile. Everyone had to bring his or her own food and drink, but when you left at the end of the evening, there was a bowl by the door in order for you to put in a contribution. Seeing as you brought your own refreshment, this was remuneration for using her premises. Once again, I was expected to pay rent for sitting on someone's settee.

There were barn dances that took place outside of Friday Folk. One was actually set in a real barn on a farm. The owners had cleared out the hay and had mucked out the manure as best they could, and strung a few fairy lights around the place. It was very nice. I wasn't bothered too much about the smell. It was better than the whiff coming from some of my dancing partners. The only trouble was that to get to any of these dances outside of St. Albans, I had to get a lift. This was a good excuse for some of the men who fancied me as they thought that it was their chance to get off with me. Luckily for me I could take Julie with me as my chaperone. Not that that always put them off.

One day nervous Stewart had given us both a lift to a dance and on the way back home, he plucked up the courage to go one step further. He said that he would drop Julie off, and then he would take me to show me how he had decorated his flat. I didn't want that. He may as well have said come up and see my etchings. He was just slowing down to drop Julie off when I said, 'Oh, Julie and I would love to come and see your flat'. Well he was completely thrown at this, and too nervous to say anything about it, so off we all went to see Stuarts decorating, while he pretended to be enjoying himself. Good old Julie. I call her my rottweiller. She kept everyone at bay.

Another person that would have liked to 'get to know me' a bit better, was Richard, he of round body and apple face. One day he came up to me and offered me a lift home from a function and I said, 'Oh yes, Julie and I would love a lift home, thank you'. Naturally, I wanted my sister to have a lift home but also I wanted someone to help keep these men at arms length. Of course, he couldn't say anything about giving us both a lift, so took us home. Once back at my flat, he asked me if I would go out with him the following night. Thinking on my feet I said, 'Oh no, Julie and I can't make it tomorrow', and Julie picked up on it and also said, 'Sorry no, I can't make it tomorrow'. To which Richard turned to Julie and said in an irritated voice, 'I wasn't asking you, I was asking Susan'.

Brian, the man I used to dance the last Polka with at the barn dances, was probably the best of a bad lot. He was quite podgy and very pompous. Again, he had a big car and a very expensive house, and was the chief accountant at British Aerospace. He had more personality than my other 'suitors', (not too difficult to achieve), and he seemed to wash more. He asked me if I would go to a concert with him at The Barbican in London. I agreed to it as he wasn't a bad chap, although as I said, a bit pompous. He came round to my flat and brought some crudités with him. Only someone like Brian would bring crudités on a date. He said that he would leave them there and we could eat them when we got back. I was quite naïve and agreed. He wasn't silly though. It was a good excuse to come back to my flat.

Anyway, we went to the concert and had a nice time. We got on reasonably well and talked about all manner of things. When we got back to my flat, ostensibly to eat his crudités

, he started telling me how I would make him a good wife. How I was just the right sort of person that could entertain his business colleagues and that I was very attractive and presentable. He said it didn't matter if I couldn't do things, because he said that he would cook and he would do this, that and the other, as long as he could have me. He had it all worked out. Then he started forcing himself on me, and was kissing and groping me, his hands wandering everywhere. He was getting more and more carried away with himself. Unfortunately, I never had my 'rottweiller' to protect me, so I had to become forceful and told him to leave. The crudités were nice though.

I still saw him at the barn dances, but I was very cool towards him. It wasn't long before he found someone else, though. She was a very attractive woman and probably fitted the bill for Brian as a future entertainer of his friends. She must have thought so too, as she eventually moved in with him.

Twice a year, Oakland's Horticultural College would hold a big barn dance. It was in the grounds of this college that the man exposed himself to me while I was at school. This was an easy venue for Julie and me to get to, and therefore we didn't need a lift from the likes of Brian, Stuart or Richard. Dad could drop us off and then pick us up after. On retrospect, I think I may have preferred Brian and co. As you can imagine, it was rather embarrassing for us to be in our twenties, having our dad drop us off for a dance and then return later to pick us up, as if we were ten year olds going to a friend's birthday party.

This particular dance was around Christmas time. It was very cold outside, and all the windows were frosted up. Towards the end of the evening, someone outside was wiping the frost off the windows and peering in. One window at a time, this mysterious visitor would scrape away the frost and gaze in, frightening the life out of anybody that happened to be looking in that direction. I remember one woman say, 'Oh, look. It's the ghost of Christmas past'.

Julie and I ignored this spectre of the night, having a suspicious feeling we knew who it was. A short time later, we were all in the middle of the floor about to start a dance, when we heard 'Clip clop, clip clop'. Everyone looked towards the noise to see Dad wandering across the stage in front of the band, oblivious to all the lights, cables and in fact musicians, dressed in his old gardening overalls and flat cap. He looked like someone who had escaped from a mental hospital. He started shouting at the top of his voice, like some deranged town crier, 'SUSAN. JULIE. HAS ANYONE SEEN MY DAUGHTERS'?

Someone said, 'What's that tramp doing on the stage? Is he part of the act'? Julie and I just looked at each other and wished the ground would open up.

The headquarters for barn dancing is Cecil Sharp House, in Regents Park, London. Every so often we would go there for a dance, but of course we would have to get a lift for these events. Despite all the bad experiences I had had from previous lifts, I wasn't going to let that stop me going to a barn dance. Therefore, I accepted a lift from nervous Stuart. He was nearly wetting himself with excitement. As he was driving along, he was so excited with the fact that I was sitting next to him, that he didn't notice that the car in front of us had stopped. He ploughed straight into the back of it and the car behind ploughed into us.

Thankfully, no one was hurt, but poor old Stuart's car was crunched up like a concertina. Nevertheless, even though he only had half a car, that wasn't going to put Stuart off. He was still determined to give me a lift to London then back again to my flat. This was his big chance; he wasn't going to blow it. Consequently, we creaked and groaned in this bashed in Metro to Cecil Sharp House and later back to St. Albans. Unfortunately for Stuart, I was only interested in getting a lift, so once we got back to my flat, I said, 'Well, thank you very much Stuart. Goodnight', and went in. I left him to creak and groan back home alone.

New Years Eve was always important to me. I had always been used to going out to celebrate it, whether it was round a neighbour's house when I lived at home, or something that was organised by the Westminster Missionaries. It always felt wrong to stay in on New Year, and so I would always try to do something, if I was well enough.

This particular year there was no local dances going on, but Dana, Kathy, Julie and I had heard of a barn dance in a church hall at Mill Hill. This was called a Circassian Circle barn dance. Well, that meant nothing to us. As far as we were concerned, a barn dance was a barn dance. The four of us turned up already feeling a bit sorry for ourselves because we were four women on our own and at our age we should have had boyfriends or husbands to escort us to places.

When we walked into the hall, we immediately felt out of place. Everyone there was wearing coordinated clothing. The men wore white shirts and black trousers and the women wore black tops and white skirts. It was like a uniform. We had just turned up in our usual barn dancing dresses. When the dancing started, the uniformity carried on. These people were very serious about their dancing. No one put a foot wrong. It was as if they were competing for an Olympic medal. Of course, the four of us didn't know the dances anywhere near as well as these people. We were going back when we should have gone forwards, do-see-do-ing when we should have been stripping the willow and taking our partner when we should have been taking someone else's. All the while, these people were getting more and more annoyed with us. They kept coming up to us and saying, 'Don't you know you're doing it all wrong? You're spoiling the whole evening'. We should have been enjoying ourselves, but instead we wished we hadn't come.

Just as we thought it couldn't get any worse, I looked across the room to spot a beckoning finger. 'Come hither' was there! As soon as he spotted us his face lit up, this was his big chance. Here were four unattached females that he could conduct through the evening. Having nothing to lose, and getting fed up with being told off by the people we were partnering, we all circled round Come Hither and danced with him. Well, his finger worked overtime that night, as he hithered and dithered. He must have thought all his Christmases had come at once.

Years later, on another New Years Eve, I went to another barn dance miles from St. Albans, and by coincidence bumped into nervous Stuart. He told me that the Friday Folk was still going strong, and most of the old members still went. Come Hither, Richard, Abdu, they were all still going, still trying to find someone. I found that rather sad and was glad I was now out of it.

Back on the work front, I eventually got a clerical job through Blue Arrow. It was in a company called SeaCare International, which was an insurance company for seafarers. I was still a temp, but working full time. This job was monotonous and repetitive, and it did my depression no good at all.

I went to see my G.P Dr. Gorton, and he said, 'Well Susan, you're getting more depressed and less able to cope with life. None of the medication I have given you has worked, and the side affects are making you worse'. I had to agree. 'I have a suggestion', he said. 'How about if I refer you to the Maudsley Hospital as an inpatient? This is a world-renowned teaching hospital for psychological problems. Some of the finest psychiatrists in the country work there.'

Well, it was true that I had come to the end of the line and needed something to help me. Conversely, I was a nervous about going into hospital.

'It'll be alright', he reassured me, 'you'll only go in for two to six weeks. The maximum will be six weeks, but it probably won't be as long as that'. He went on, 'They have specialists working there, and they'll be able to try out different medications on you. They can monitor your progress and fine-tune the drugs until they find the right thing for you. They will be able to sort out your eating disorder, the depression, in fact all your problems. When you come out you will be able to live a normal life again'.

This sounded too good to be true. I was going to be cured. I didn't like the idea of going into hospital, but on the other hand, I desperately wanted to be well. I plucked up my courage and said to him, 'Yes please. Put the process in motion. I'll go there'.

That was in May 1988. My life was now more or less on hold. I wasn't working, and led a very limited life at home, although I still went to Friday Folk. I would go for a walk in the afternoons if I felt well enough. But I wasn't getting better. I had ups and downs, but truthfully more downs than ups.

Time wore on and things were getting steadily worse, and I hadn't heard anything about my admittance to hospital. One day at the beginning of August, I was having a particularly bad morning. The depression was black and I knew that I just couldn't carry on the way I was. Life just wasn't worth living. I decided that I had had enough and so I went to a phone box to phone the consultant's office at the Maudsley. In my naïve way, I hadn't realised that an ordinary person like me didn't phone consultants. I know now that usually if you phone a consultant, or even an ordinary doctor, you get through to an overworked receptionist who might put you through to the office cleaner. Fortunately I didn't know this and as luck would have it, got straight through to the consultant's secretary. I spoke to her and tried to explain how things were and how desperate I was and I broke down and cried on the phone. I must have made an impact with her, as she told me that the consultant, Dr. Noble, wasn't there at the moment, but if I were to phone back at half past four I could speak to him.

I duly phoned back and, despite how busy he must have been, miraculously he spoke to me. I told him between sobs how things were with me, and he said, 'Well, I haven't actually seen a referral for you, but you sound in a pretty bad way. So I'll give you an appointment to see me next week'. I thanked him very much. With hindsight, I wouldn't have thanked him, or even have called him in the first place. That phone call booked my place in hell.

I went the following week with Dad to see this specialist. He said that obviously I was in a bad way and desperately needed help. He said that I had been suffering for too long, and trying to carry the load alone. He said that the best thing for me to do was to come in as an inpatient, and they would do their best to put things right. I was admitted to the Maudsley Hospital on August Bank Holiday weekend 1988. The nightmare begins.

THE MAUDSLEY

This was to be the darkest chapter in my life so far. I was going to call this chapter 'The Day the Sun Died', because as far as I was concerned, that's precisely how it felt the day I walked into to the Maudsley. I had no choice but to admit myself as an inpatient. I was not coping at all in my flat; in fact, I was spending more and more time at home with Mum and Dad, but in the deepest of depressions and desperately unhappy. I may have been very naïve, but I firmly believed that this would be my salvation.

The Maudsley Hospital in Denmark Hill, London, is a big, dark, imposing building. It is also a renowned teaching hospital and some of the most eminent Psychiatrists and Psychologists lecture there. I saw no eminent Psychiatrists or Psychologists during my stay. The part of the hospital I was on was well away from anyone eminent. Of course, I wasn't to know that when I arrived. I was very apprehensive about going in, but I was also full of hope that this place was going to get me better. My doctor had told me that. At that stage in my life, I believed anything a doctor told me. After all, they're the experts.

Dad accompanied me to the hospital and we walked arm in arm along the bleak, austere corridors. Every so often there would be a locked door with a little porthole in the middle with safety glass inset. I had never seen the inside of a prison, except on television, but this was how I imagined it. These were the wards. We went up two flights of stone stairs and arrived at my ward. The ward assigned to me consisted of two groups of patients, with a consultant in charge of each group. One group contained people suffering mainly from eating disorders, notably Anorexia Nervosa, with Professor Russell as the consultant in charge. The other general group, which included me, had Dr. Noble as the consultant in charge.

As a number of the patients were thought to be dangerous, either to themselves or to others, the security on most of the wards was high. I was to be locked in with potentially violent people. That was a very frightening aspect.

We rang the bell to the ward, and an orderly came to let us in. I noticed that dangling from her belt was a huge set of keys. That reinforced the notion of prison in my mind. The other thing that struck me was the dishevelled sight of the orderlies. They wore for the most part, tatty old jeans and stained sweatshirts. I thought at first that they were patients. Even the trained nurses dressed the same, albeit perhaps a bit cleaner.

The other thing that struck me was how few trained nurses there were on the ward. There was always one SRN, who ran the ward. There was also one junior nurse, and about five orderlies. There were about 35 patients on my ward, so seven staff members gave a 5 to 1 ratio, which sounds good. Nevertheless, when you consider that many of the patients were on 24-hour suicide watch, which took away one member staff each, the ratio wasn't that good.

Many of the orderlies were students but a large number were foreigners who could hardly speak English. I wonder if many of them could have got a job anywhere else. In fact, later on during my stay, I was given a key worker who was supposed to find the underlying cause of my problems and help me over come them. She was so bad at speaking English that unless I learned how to speak Filipino, we were going to be in a quandary.

The orderly led Dad and me through this ward to where my bed was going to be. She told me that this was the anorexics eating area and dorm. There was a long trestle table in the middle of this room, where the anorexics had their meals. She went away and a male orderly came up to me and took my bag. He emptied all the contents out onto the bed and went through every item. I felt ashamed as every intimate possession was scrutinised, from underwear to sanitary towels. He performed the search in a very cold, dispassionate, way. They obviously did hundreds of these searches every year and it showed. There was no emotion, no feeling, no compassion, nothing. What made it worse for me was that they didn't even have the consideration to have a female orderly do it. They were looking for razors, knives, tablets, laxatives; in fact, any means of killing yourself or any means of getting rid of food. Then a female 'warder' came and gave me an intimate body search. I know they have to be careful and that they were only doing their job, but I felt like a criminal. I felt so humiliated, so mortified, in fact so ashamed at what my life had come to, through no fault of my own, that I broke down and cried.

After the search, she told me that I had to leave the dorm, still with my possessions strewn all over the bed, as it was time for the anorexics to have their meal. The staff allowed nobody in during meal times. They would have a trained nurse stationed at one end of the table, forcing these people to eat. After the meals, the patients had to lie on the beds for an hour. This was to prevent them vomiting up the food, or using laxatives or even exercising the meal away.

As one of these beds was to be mine, and I could not use it during these times, it was going to be like a time-share. The meal times went on for as long as it took the anorexics to eat their food, which could take three hours. Moreover, they got six meals a day: breakfast, a mid morning snack, lunch, afternoon snack, evening meal and supper. In reality, that meant I could only use dorm at night to sleep.

Dad and I came out of the anorexic dorm and we went into the only other place available, which was the day room. It was now time for Dad to leave, so I said a tearful goodbye and the orderly let him out and locked the door. I waved to him through the porthole in the door and watched him walk away. The realisation hit me then like a wave. I was a prisoner. I came here of my own free will, but I couldn't get out. What had I done to deserve this?

I went back to the day room and looked around. What a God-awful place it was. It was a large room with plastic chairs around the outside, with a large TV on a stand. There was a horrible, grimy carpet, that I'm sure had a pattern on it at one time, but now the pattern was made up with stubbed out cigarettes, coffee stains and other unrecognisable gunge. The walls had at one time been a magnolia colour, which was now magnolia and filth. You wouldn't find the shade on a colour chart in a DIY shop. At first, I didn't realise that there were windows in the day room. On closer inspection, I found out that there were, but they were hard to see through due to the layers of accumulated grime. Hanging from the ceiling were strip lights, and hanging from the strip lights were cobwebs containing an assortment of dead insects.

There were a number of people in the ward who were very ill and whose personal hygiene left a lot to be desired, and who sat on the chairs all day. Consequently, the chairs were dirty and soiled. It was not a very welcoming place to sit. The general environment began to demoralize me from the beginning.

Obviously being a lock up ward in a mental hospital, there were people that you didn't want to sit next to. Some very seriously ill and sometimes dangerous people would threaten you or go crazy and rip the curtains down, and smash the place up. Suffice to say you did anything to avoid sitting in the day room. Nevertheless, if that was the only place available, then you had no choice.

That first day, after Dad had gone, I was standing in the day room looking out of one of the windows, after first scraping off some of the grime, and took in the wonderful view it gave; horrible patches of scrub and concrete, which was all fenced off. This served as an exercise yard for the patients. Further on from this were yet more drab concrete walls, which led to another part of the hospital. There were also tunnelled walkways that connected different parts of the building. If you were not depressed when you came in, you certainly were after looking out of the window.

I started to cry. My key worker, Chris, came over. He said to me, 'Well, what's the matter with you then?' Well, I thought, you're on the ball. He was supposed to know what the matter with me was. How was I to explain? Where would I begin? Before I could start to tell him what was wrong, he said, 'Well, I would try and get out of here if I were you'.

What was I to do, dig a tunnel? I couldn't believe what I was hearing. I believed that nurses and doctors were there to help you, and that they were knowledgeable and switched on. He was as thick as they came. As he wandered off to do whatever it was he did for a living, (sleep probably) and left me to cry, another man came up to me. He was an anorexic, and a seemingly educated man. 'Are you a new nurse?' he asked me.

'No', I said between sobs, 'I'm a new patient'. That's when it really hit me, when I realised that I had hit rock bottom. The tears were now streaming down my face. The man looked at me with kindly eyes and said, 'Tell me what's wrong. You look like there's nothing wrong with you'.

I tried explaining to this man, who was the nicest person I had met up to now, that I was suffering from depression, because I didn't know how to explain the myriad of problems that I had. I can't remember that man's name, and I didn't really get to know him, as he was about to be discharged from the hospital. I believe he was a television producer or at least in television production. However later on, in a strange quirk of fate, he was to be a catalyst in a main period in my life.

Professor Gerald Russell, the consultant in charge of the eating disorder clinic, was the first person to bring any organised regime in Britain for the treatment for anorexia. His view of anorexia was quite simplistic. Anorexics starved themselves until their body weight was so low that they died. Therefore, if he fed them up enough, they would live.

Of course, this was true. While on his ward, the anorexics didn't die from being underweight, but then, they weren't cured either. As soon as they got to a reasonable weight, he would discharge them back into the community, where they possibly would die. The regime was akin to fattening turkeys up for Christmas. During the six months I was there, I witnessed dozens of these people returning to the ward, after they had starved themselves again. You see, the problem with anorexia is that not eating is just a symptom of the illness. There is a reason that they don't eat. Whatever their rationale is, they believe themselves to be fat. Fattening them up is not going to make their problems go away. As soon as they leave the hospital, they will starve themselves once more, sometimes to death.

Medical research has since established that the underlying cause for people thinking themselves to be fat has to be rooted out. They should have counselling to help them to overcome the problem themselves, so that they will eat of their own free will, and mentally adjust to putting on weight. Anorexics fear eating. They already think of themselves as fat. If you then force them to eat six meals a day, that would only add to the terror of their phobia. In their eyes, they are now obese.

From talking to patients, both during my six months on the ward and then afterwards as an outpatient, plus my contact with various anorexics in later years, I concluded that there wasn't one person who was cured as part of this regime.

Those of us who were not anorexics had our meals in a separate dining room off the ward. We had to line up, with a 'warder' at the front and one at the back. The warder at the front selected a key from the large assortment on her chain, and unlocked the door to let us out. We then marched single file to the main dining room, which was down two flights of stairs. It was like being in a chain gang. The only things that were missing were the guard tower and spotlights.

All around the wards and dining area were panic buttons, which the staff activated whenever things got out of control. These panic buttons let out an awful wailing noise. The sirens would also go off if someone escaped from the hospital. Once triggered, staff would run from all parts of the hospital to help their colleagues.

We all had to wait outside the dining hall, to be let in a few at a time. Once in, you picked up your plastic tray and walked along a counter, behind which stood the surly kitchen staff who served you. You could then choose, from a row of containers with their diverse selection of slop, the least disgusting meal. Once you had your meal, you went to find a place to eat it at one of the trestle tables. All around were these warders, for that is how I saw them, watching you eat. It couldn't have been more like a prison. Everyone who was not anorexic ate in this canteen, including all the violent patients. There was no segregation, so you would sit there trying to eat your slop, and across the room someone would be ranting, raving, and smashing up the place before making a bid for freedom. These would be escapees would then be felled by half a dozen orderlies, given a 'liquid cosh' and taken back to the ward. The liquid cosh was used on a number of occasions. On one occasion a man didn't want to take his medication, as he said it was affecting him adversely. The orderlies held him down with his arms pinned behind his back and gave him a liquid cosh. They then carried him back to his bed and administered the drug. So much for free will, I thought.

On this first night, I saw a group of men who were in the process of becoming women. Having led a very innocent life, I had never heard of transsexuals before this. I don't think the operation was commonplace in the mid eighties, and the whole idea was hardly spoken about outside, certainly not in my circles. Some of these men/women were very distressed. They were in the aftermath of the operation and a lot of them seemed to be having a bad time coming to terms with it.

There would be people who would have weird conversations with themselves and everyone else. You dared not look at some people, who seemed extremely vicious. If they caught you, they would lunge at you screaming, 'What are you looking at'?

The noise was unbelievable. It was like a bear garden. There were people who were right off their heads who should have been in a segregated part. The aggression and hostility of some of those people was terrifying. Although I knew that the nurses were around, it didn't take long for my trust in them to diminish. For the most part, they just stood there with their arms folded talking to each other, only getting involved when they absolutely had to. There was always a desperate shortage of staff, which was not surprising considering the work involved. The hospital relied heavily on agency staff, who were either foreign and couldn't speak the language, or else just lazy, apathetic individuals who were not interested in working, and certainly not interested in helping the likes of me. Some were just blatantly cruel and sadistic.

The noise, the threats, and indeed the level of intimidation are indescribable. I had never known fear like it, before or since. Never mind, I thought, it's only for a fortnight and I'll be out of here, cured. I realise now how naïve I was.

When the evening came, the orderlies allowed me to go to my bed, now that all the meals were over.

The metal beds had a small locker next to them and about 18 inches between each bed. There was just enough room for a curtain to go round, although the staff did not allow a patient to do this. You were under observation all the time. The night staff then came on. An Irish woman, whom they must have forgotten when feelings were distributed, was in charge. She was just as cold and sadistic as they came. She came in and snarled at us, 'Come on. I want you lot to bed. I don't want any trouble from any of you tonight'.

With that, they marched us into the washrooms. If you went to the toilet, the doors had to remain open. If you closed the door, they would kick it open watch you go to the toilet. I can't think of anything more humiliating. After going to the toilet, you then went to have a wash and clean your teeth. They allocated three minutes for that. If you had forgotten anything, like your toothbrush, you could not go back and get it. I'm convinced that convicted criminals got better treatment. I had done nothing wrong. My only crime was that I was ill.

I got into bed, with thoughts of the day swirling around my head. Why me? I thought, what have I done to deserve this life? I cried myself to sleep. I tell you now, if tears were pound coins, over the years I could have paid off the third world debt.

I woke up with a start in the dead of night. It was pitch black, and I looked up to see this person looming over me. I let out an almighty scream, waking up the whole ward. I thought my time was up, that someone was going to kill me. Then this woman said, 'Oh, it's all right dear, I didn't mean any harm. I just wanted you to tell me, does my stomach look big?'

This was an anorexic lady called Pauline. Someone called out, 'It's all right Pauline, your stomach's not big. Go back to bed'.

It seemed that this was a regular occurrence with Pauline. There really was no harm in her, but you can imagine my fright at seeing someone coming towards me in the middle of the night, after all the events I had witnessed.

That then was my first night. The morning didn't bode much better. Around 7am, the whole ward was woken up, but not to singing nightingales, or even Florence Nightingales. We were all forcefully shaken awake by the orderlies, who seemed to enjoy doing it. I later found out that, as many patients were on various potent drugs, the staff had to shake them to get them out of their almost comatose state. Mind you, the staff didn't try to find out who was on the drugs and who wasn't. We were all treated the same. If any patient didn't get up after being so gently woken, then they would have their mattress pulled out from under them, which meant that the prisoner, sorry, patient fell onto the springs underneath. In addition, if the staff felt that a patient was spending too long on their bed during the day, they would remove the mattress altogether and lock it away. Some of those patients were so sedated with the drugs they were taking, that they were desperate for sleep. I watched many just fall down on to the bedsprings and go out for the count.

There were about thirty-five patients on my ward, but only three sinks for female patients, which was the reason we only had three minutes in which to wash ourselves. Again, an orderly oversaw all the ablutions, including going to the toilet. Having had your wash, you went back to get dressed. You had to make your own bed, before leaving for the day room. I tried not to forget anything I needed from the dorm, because I would not be allowed to go back to get it.

Then it was a repeat of the day before, wherein the nurses closed the doors to the dorm, as the anorexics filed in. The rest of us lined up to be escorted down to the dining hall for breakfast. After breakfast, we came back on the ward and the patients who were able, went to the sheltered workshop for occupational therapy. Occupational therapy was from 10 to 12, then after lunch, 2 to 4. You did wonderfully fulfilling jobs such as packing nails, packing sponges or packing toothbrushes. They didn't expect you to do this for nothing, mind you. Oh no. They paid you the princely sum of ten pence an hour. If you worked especially hard you were held up as an example to all the others; 'You too could be like this', sort of thing. If you worked overtime, you could clear £2.50 a week. Unfortunately, that wasn't really enough with which to bribe a guard. Those patients who were unable to do this highflying work, or were under assessment, (as I was for the first two weeks) would sit in the day room and watch daytime television, so anyone who did not have depression soon would have.

I very rarely saw a doctor, unless it was a trainee, and I certainly never saw my consultant. I doubt if a consultant ever saw a patient unless he was playing golf with them. After being in the hospital for a fortnight, I had the privilege of seeing the trainee doctor, who was Spanish. She was studying psychiatry before going back home to practise. She should have studied English before coming here. It was like having a conversation with Manuel from Fawlty Towers.

Jumping ahead a bit, I saw this woman on and off for the six months that I was an inpatient there. Towards the end of my treatment, she told me that she was pleased that she had cured my obsession with smashing windows. Well, I had never smashed a window in my life, although I was sorely tempted now. She was mistaking me with another girl on the ward, Yvonne, who was also suffering with depression, and who used to vent her anger by smashing windows.

Try as I might, I couldn't get through to this Spanish trainee idiot that it was someone else that smashed windows, not me. She was adamant that she had cured me and that was that. You can imagine the confidence that filled me with. She was treating me for something that I never had, and taking the credit for curing me of it. Anyway, that was at the end of my time there, and by then, I had come to expect that sort of incompetence.

Day to day life on the ward was very boring. You would expect it to be regimented, which in a way I would have preferred, but in fact once the staff had done what they had to do, for example escort you to meals and dish out drugs, you were left to your own devices. There were long stretches of time to fill in this abhorrent environment. I could see why packing screws would be regarded as an exciting option to some people.

Obviously, being on the anorexic dorm was quite restrictive. Therefore, I requested to move and they transferred me to a glorified alcove in the corridor. There were four beds, separated by a half wall. There was one major drawback to this alcove, in that the strip lights stayed on all night. That was because it was part of the corridor that the nurses used to get to the anorexic dorm and the linen cupboard. Therefore, I didn't really get any sleep there. I'm sure dictators from third world countries used to come to the Maudsley to get tips on torture.

The advantage of moving to this alcove was that at least I could get to my bed space during the day. There was no extra privacy, as there was no door, but on the plus side, there was quite a good view out of the window. Whereas the view out of the other windows was just concrete and scrubland, out of this window was a wonderful panoramic view of London. You could see the Post Office Tower and St. Thomas's Hospital and the Thames. I could imagine the hustle and bustle of city life, with people going about their business enjoying themselves. How I envied them their normality. It was all just a thickness of glass away, but unlike Alice, I couldn't go the other side of the glass to join in. I might as well have been in prison.

My roommates in the alcove were two girls called Yasmin and Clare, who became great friends with each other. Clare had at one time been a staff nurse at St. Thomas' Hospital, but was now in the Maudsley suffering from Anorexia. In keeping with Professor Russell's' policy, Clare went through the regime of being fattened up and then returned into the community. She had already gone through this process once and was back in the hospital after nearly starving herself to death.

Claire had also started self-harming and had lacerated all her arms and wrists. I once saw her arms and had never seen anything like it before. There must have been 40 lacerations on each arm. There wasn't a millimetre of space between the cuts. Her wrists had bandages on where she had slashed them, covering up the stitches. She was now on the general ward so that they could get to grips with her problems, as if they were different now from what they had been. They couldn't seem to understand that it was the same problem.

As far as I could see, Professor Russell treated anorexia as people who just couldn't eat, as if it was a phobia, akin to being afraid of heights. He thought that if he fattened the patients up, all their problems would be over. Nothing could be further from the truth. Anorexia Nervosa is just a symptom, a by-product. Getting to the root cause as to why the patient won't eat, is the first step in solving that. Clare was one of many anorexics that I knew that used the entrance to the hospital like a revolving door. They were not really a feather in Professor Russell's cap.

The other girl, Yasmin, suffered from paranoid schizophrenia and when I first moved into the alcove, she would spend all her time curled up in a ball surrounded by soft toys. Yasmin was Asian and her parents were both non-medical professors. Her mother would come and visit her, but her father refused. He couldn't accept that his daughter was in a place like this. After a while, Yasmin's medication started to work, and she became less afraid of people and started to relate to them rather than to soft toys. Both Yasmin and Clare left hospital before me and I lost touch with both of them, although I did find out from someone who knew Yasmin that she became ill again later on. I don't know what became of Clare. I hope she is all right.

Fortunately, the hospital only kept me in over one weekend, which was the first weekend I was there. I remember that Mum, Dad and Julie came to visit me that first weekend. I had managed to manipulate the Spanish trainee doctor into letting me go home every other weekend. Most of my problems stemmed around not being able to cope in my flat on my own. Therefore, the medical staff decided that I would need time on my own in the flat working on the various tasks that they set for me. They didn't give me any coping strategies or tips. They would say, 'Try and hoover the living room, or clean the bathroom or something'. At least it meant that I was out the place for a couple of days.

Julie would come to my flat Friday evening, and we would go to Friday Folk. As far as anyone could see, it was business as usual. The Mass centre and Friday folk all carried on as normal during the time I was in the Maudsley.

I have long known that people are afraid of mental illness. It's stigma by association. They are afraid that it may be catching or that if someone has a mental illness then they are going to attack you with an axe. Statistics show that one in four people will suffer from some form of mental illness in their life. For most people, these are transient states. For example, many people get depression if a loved one dies or they are made redundant. Postnatal depression is another good example. Sadly, for many others, the problem will last a lifetime. They have to try to live with it the best they can. Of course, some can't live with it.

Mental illnesses are some of the least understood conditions in society. Because of this, many people face prejudice and discrimination in their everyday lives. I have experienced this first hand. Instead of being a person, you become your illness. If a diagnosis becomes a label, it can be very damaging. For example, instead of seeing someone as a parent, writer, or teacher who has schizophrenia, that person is labelled a schizophrenic, as though this diagnosis sums him or her up. It's important to remember that having a mental illness is not someone's fault, it s not a sign of weakness, and it's not something to be ashamed of.

Getting back to my weekends out, on the Saturday I would try to conquer whatever my particular fear or problem was, be it hoovering or dusting, whatever. Sometimes Julie would be with me for moral support, but not all the time. On Sunday, I would go to Mum and Dad's for dinner, then in the afternoon would head back to Denmark Hill and my five star accommodation in the Maudsley. Along with letting me out at weekends, I was also free to leave the ward during the day the rest of the week. Only the anorexics stayed under lock and key, along with anyone who the staff considered a risk to themselves or a threat to others.

If you were canny enough, you could work the system in your favour. The staff didn't really know or even care what was going on, as long as they had an easy life. To that end, I escaped work detail. I used to wait until after breakfast, then queue up with all the others that were going to the workshops to pack screws. I would leave the ward with them but then carry on out the main door, go to Camberwell, and walk round the shops. The anorexics and others, who were not allowed off the ward, would give me a shopping list of things that they wanted, and I would bring them back.

Also at that time, I was still abusing laxatives. That was how I controlled my weight. Of course, the hospital didn't know that. If they had found out, I would have been put under Professor Russell's 'care'. Therefore, I smuggled in the laxatives, as my bag wasn't checked. Once on the ward I would keep them hidden in my underwear in my locker, or more often than not, in my purse which I kept with me at all times. Periodically there were searches. There were some potentially violent cases on the ward and some self-harmers, so the staff would search for weapons. There were also drug addicts on the ward so the staff would also search for drugs. Having said all that, the security was nevertheless quite lax, as the majority of the orderlies were apathetic and lethargic. Therefore, a lot of illicit contraband came in undetected.

If I didn't go to the shops then I would walk round Ruskin Park, which was a lovely, tranquil place, opposite the hospital. I really enjoyed doing that. It was like stepping out of hell and into the Garden of Eden. A couple of times Dad visited me, and we walked together round the park. There was a library in Ruskin Park, and in the winter when it got dark early I would go in, (with the tramps and alcoholics), and just sit there. I wasn't mentally capable of taking anything in that I read, as the drugs had all but sedated me, by I would pretend to read. I would do anything rather than go back to the ward.

Occasionally, during my promenade around Ruskin Park, I would meet up with a man who was a patient in a ward below me that I first met during a relaxation class. That's where a lady with a tape player would play classical music and we would all lie around relaxing to it. It was like being back at infant school. I was waiting for her to tell us all to be trees or butterflies or something.

Anyway, this man also hated packing nails, so he too would make a break for it and go for a walk around the park. I preferred being on my own, but occasionally it was nice to have a bit of company. He told me that he used to spend his days hiding underneath his bed as he was trying to come to terms with being a homosexual. I saw him a few months later when I was an outpatient, standing in a supermarket queue French kissing another man. I presume he had come to terms with it.

As well as the relaxation class, another aspect to the 'recovery program' in the Maudsley was an anxiety management class. There were about a dozen of us altogether, all handpicked from different wards, whom the staff felt were intelligent enough to talk through our problems and by doing so, benefit from it. One patient from this group was a middle-aged bespectacled man with a beard, who had an alcohol problem. He told everyone that he quelled his anxiety with drink. The group was a bit like alcoholics anonymous, in that everyone took a turn in telling the rest of the group what their problem was. I spoke about my anxiety, and what came to the fore was my low self-esteem and how I tried to quell my anxiety with food. I told of my exaggerated concern over what I imagine other people thought about me.

The upshot was they decided that because of my low self-image combined with my anxiety, the answer was exercise. As a result, they told me to go to the local swimming pool, along with the bearded alcoholic. Naturally, I had to change into a swimming costume, which I hadn't done since I was a teenager, playing 'Ball o on the beach' with Dad and Julie. This was not such a good idea. Firstly, I don't like my body, (I still don't to this day), and so putting on a swimming costume made me cringe with embarrassment. Secondly, I'm not a very good swimmer and thirdly I don't like water. That is not a good combination of phobias to have when you go swimming.

Nevertheless, I was prepared to do anything to try to help myself. I gently lowered myself into the pool and started swimming up and down in the shallow end. However, this was a public pool and it was full of yobs splashing each other and me and making as much noise as they could. They could see how frightened I was, so they did it some more. I persevered for about half an hour, but I hated every minute of it. I finally had enough, got out of the pool, had a shower, and changed. I never went back.

I escaped from the work detail as often as I could but after a while even the most lethargic of orderlies realised that instead of diligently going to the workshop, I was walking round the park or going to the shops. So, rather than being shot at dawn, off to the workshop I went.

The workshop was reminiscent of a large Nissen hut. It was a very dark place, (as was most of the hospital) with high windows that let hardly any light in. The lighting, such as it was, shone down from circular metal shades up on the ceiling, similar to war time prison camps. Some people liked going to this workshop. In fact, my key worker told me I would 'only' be able to go three afternoons a week, as the rest of the time it was full up. I tried not to smile.

The jobs in this place changed from day to day. One day you may be packing toothbrushes, the next day sponges or nails. You had to count out so many into a pack, before passing it to someone else to be sealed. Sometimes it was simple assembly work, wherein you would attach two things with a nut and bolt that was then going to go somewhere else to make a bigger thing. I never knew nor cared what the things were. All I knew was that it was soul destroying, mind numbing work. I likened it to prisoners sewing mailbags.

I cried whenever I was in the workshop, as I realised what I had come to. Whenever I thought I had hit rock bottom, there was something else around the corner.

Prior to my stay at the Maudsley, I went to see a group of people who took over from the Westminster Missionaries, who called themselves The Upper Room Prayer Group. Most of the people that I knew from the Westminster Missionaries had long gone, so I didn't really know these people very well. Nevertheless, I phoned the two members that ran the group, a girl called Sheila and a man called Dave Payne, because I knew that they ran group homes. Because I couldn't cope in my flat on my own, I wondered if I could move into one of the shared houses, and live with them. I knew it wouldn't be an ideal solution, as I didn't like sharing due to some of the bad experiences I'd had in the past, but I saw it as a possibility. Unfortunately, the shared houses were more like religious retreats. You know the kind of thing, work, rest and pray. All the housemates had full time jobs and shared the bills. I had no job and subsequently couldn't pay my way, but apart from that, they didn't really want someone with a mental illness in one of their homes. So, that put paid to that.

The medical staff at the Maudsley mooted a similar idea to mine. They decided that if I couldn't survive in a self-contained place, my best option would be to move into a home run by The Richmond Fellowship. These are hostels up and down the country for people who are too psychologically ill to cope alone and need the support of others. It was true that I found it hard to manage on my own, but at the same time, I didn't want to live in a hostel. I had seen these places before and they had been dirty and foul smelling and I would have hated living in one. I didn't regard myself as that far gone. I would have been no better off than if I stayed at the Maudsley. I also knew that once I had moved into one of those places, then that would be a point of no return. I would never get out.

I discussed this with my family and luckily they agreed with me that it wouldn't be a good idea for me to move into a Richmond Fellowship Hostel. I think they realised that if I did, I would be on a downward spiral from which I would never recover. We decided that one way or another, I would soldier on in my flat.

Changing the subject, perhaps this is a good time to tell you about Pauline, the lady who gave me a shock on my first night but only wanted to know if her stomach was big. Pauline was a woman in her fifties who had developed anorexia. It is quite unusual to get anorexia that late in life. She was married to a University professor, who looked not unlike Einstein, but was very dirty and scruffy, with a long beard and wild hair. He would come in and visit Pauline from time to time, and blended in very nicely with the more insalubrious of inmates. He was a typical absent-minded professor, and hardly even knew that she was there. She told me that their courting didn't amount to much more than sitting on a park bench. Having done that for about a year, he said to her, 'Well, we've been seeing each other for a year now, shall we get married?' From what I gathered from Pauline, that just about summed up their entire relationship. They somehow managed to have two boys, who were equally oblivious to their mother.

Pauline wasn't coping in the home, and the two boys and her husband treated her like a skivvy and ignored her. To them, she was simply the provider of meals and the person who did the washing and the cleaning. All this was taking its toll on Pauline, so in order for her to cope with the amount of work she had to do, she started skipping her morning coffee break. She found that if she didn't have a mid morning snack, she had more time to make the bed or do the washing up and so on. After a while, this skipping of coffee and a biscuit progressed into skipping meals. The rest of her family didn't notice, so long as they got their meals they didn't care what Pauline did. The family never sat down for a meal together, preferring to eat their meals in their bedrooms. Nobody communicated with anyone else. Her family treated her like dirt and didn't care how she was, as long as the housework was done. So Pauline stopped eating. That was the only control Pauline had left in her life.

Almost without exception, all the anorexic patients I met were very intelligent. Many were very talented and very articulate; some of them were high achievers. They could talk eloquently on a variety of subjects. Not Pauline though. I believe she had had a breakdown, and that there was more to her illness than her anorexia. She was always quite vague and simple minded. She would only really talk about the size of her stomach.

I found out that Pauline was also very religious, which interested me as I too had a strong faith. At that time, I was sleeping in the linen cupboard, (which I will come to later). Pauline would visit me there and we would read The Bible and pray together. We would then look out of the dirty windows to the massive, illuminated white cross on the Salvation Army Building opposite. We would put all our hope, trust, and faith into that cross, and all that it signified. However, I became more and more sceptical as time went on, as it seemed that my prayers were going unanswered.

That cross would shine out, supposedly signifying the love of God, lighting up everyone's life. That radiant cross became to me the paradoxical face of God, like the light in an empty fridge; in other words pointless. If God loved me, why wouldn't he help me? Why was I so ill when I prayed so hard? I was so near to this symbol of Christianity that I could almost touch it, and yet I was so far away, metaphorically, that it might as well have been on the Moon.

The doctors eventually decided that Pauline wasn't just anorexic but was also a depressive, but because she wasn't responding to treatment, they decided to give her electric shock treatment, otherwise known as electro convulsive therapy (ECT). She had a series of six treatments. After sedating her, they took her down to the treatment room where they placed electrodes on her head, with a shield in her mouth so that she wouldn't bite through her tongue. They then sent a jolt of 220 volts through her head. The word barbaric doesn't even come close to describing it.

I watched them bring Pauline back to the ward, not knowing where she was or even who she was. She would have no short-term memory for about a week. After 5 or 6 days, she would start coming back to normal, remembering who she was just in time for the next treatment. She went through this nightmare every week for 6 weeks.

The theory behind ECT is that the patient would lose their long-term memory, which is supposed to be the root cause of the problems. The hypothesis is that if the memory of the event that caused the phobia or the anxiety is wiped out, then the underlying reason for the depression has also gone, and therefore the patient will no longer have the problem. It doesn't work. The first part of the theory works in that the patient does lose his or her long-term memory. However, after a while the problems return, so the patient still has depression, is still anorexic, still has phobias, but their memory has also been destroyed.

Ernest Hemingway had ECT. He wrote, 'Well, what is the sense of ruining my head and erasing my memory, which is my capital, and putting me out of business? It was a brilliant cure but we lost the patient.' He later killed himself.

Dr. John Friedberg, a neurologist wrote, 'All ECT (electric shock) does is produce brain damage. If you want brain damage, it's your prerogative... there's no more effective way than ECT. It's more effective than a car wreck, or getting hit with a blunt instrument.'

The truth is, as with most psychiatric 'solutions', the 'treatment' is often used to make life easier on the people around the patient than to actually help the patients themselves. Certain people can be so confused, depressed, suicidal or psychotic that the mental dullness, spiritual numbness, memory loss and emotional stifling of ECT may seem better in comparison. However, it is no cure of anything and never will be.

Pauline eventually left the hospital, no better than when she arrived. Yes she had put on some weight due to the regime, but then so had most of the other anorexics. The majority of them either returned to go through it all again, or died at home of malnutrition. Even when she said goodbye to me, she still asked me if her stomach was big.

Pauline and I stayed in touch for a while, with Easter and Christmas cards. However, after a while, her letters became illegible and I couldn't even understand the gobbledegook that she had written. It seemed her brain had finally stopped functioning. I don't really know what became of Pauline; I suspect she is no longer with us. She was a lovely lady with a good heart and was a very good friend to me through the hard times. I sincerely hope that she has found Jesus, that

Jesus has found her, and that she is now in peace.

Another person I would like to tell you about is Eileen. She was on the anorexic ward, in a bed right in the corner. Eileen suffered from paranoid schizophrenia. She was a small, hunchbacked woman in her late forties or early fifties. She looked not unlike a witch with thin, bony hands, long straggly hair and very sharp features.

She wouldn't speak to anyone at first, but I made a concerted effort to get to know her. I tended to reach out to the ones who seemed to be on their own, and didn't seem to have any friends. I'm still inclined to do that to this day. I suppose it stems from my history of being shunned and being the outcast. After a while we struck up a rapport together, although she was always a bit weird. I found out that she lived in a tower block in Camberwell, but had no relatives, or at least if she did then they didn't want to know her. They put her on Haliperidal for her illness, which is a drug that makes your arms and legs shake. She led a very lonely, horrendous life, as did many of the people I met in the Maudsley.

Eileen left hospital some time before me and we did keep in touch for a while. I do know that she attempted suicide several times by drinking weed killer. One year I sent her a Christmas card and received no reply. I can only assume that one of her attempts had been successful.

There was a young girl, whose name I can't remember, who was there because she was seriously underweight. She was different to the other patients in that she believed in Professor Russell's regime. She would happily eat anything that they put in front of her. As time went on, she put on the required weight and the hospital discharged her. From what I gather, she carried on eating the same way outside the hospital. Her anorexia had turned into binge eating, which happens a lot in these cases. Unfortunately because her body was not used to eating the amount of calories she was taking in, her heart gave out. I believe a similar tragedy happened to the singer Karen Carpenter.

Another girl on the ward looked like a living skeleton. She was so thin that she could hardly walk, like a victim of a concentration camp. She weighed only four and a half stone. Her name was Angie. Angie's parents were doctors and were always pushing her to achieve and succeed.

Many experts believe that there may be a correlation between a certain style of parenting and anorexia. They argue that anorexia can develop when parents set excessively high standards of achievement or exert too much control over their children. Children of authoritative parents don't rebel. Instead, they find areas in their lives where they do have control. The main area they have control over is their eating. Eventually, these children begin to develop a distorted view of how they look. Psychological disturbances cause them to stop seeing themselves realistically, which in turn causes them to have a low self-image. Often, other peoples' references to chubbiness, pudginess, or baby fat send the signal that weight must be lost.

Bright and successful people see themselves as disgustingly fat. They feel that they have to measure up, but that they can't unless they change their body weight. Anorexia is about control; they deal with pressure by taking control of their food.

Angie's parents eventually moved away and gave her a cottage in the country where she lived alone with her dog. They just couldn't cope with her illness any more. Essentially, she would eat next to nothing but would carry out a punishing schedule of exercise each day. As undernourished as Angie was, to the extent that she could hardly stand unaided, she would push herself to walk the dog about seven miles every day. This overwhelming compulsion for hard physical exercise is a common factor amongst many anorexics. They will use any means to avoid putting on weight.

Despite Angie being on the ward for longer than the prescribed three-month period, she hardly put on any weight. She discharged herself when she was only six and a half stone. I kept in touch with her as best I could, although she would cut herself off from society from time to time. Periodically she wrote to me, although it was quite hard to understand her handwriting. It was similar to Pauline's in as much as it was frantic and disjointed, which obviously reflected her state of mind. Angie was part of the revolving door syndrome. They would find her chronically underweight; bring her back into the hospital where they would section her under the mental health act, before discharging her when her three months were up.

As with the majority of anorexics, Angie had many rituals surrounding food and exercise. She would cut her food into tiny segments, push them around her plate so many times and then chew each mouthful a set number of times. The nurses made Angie stop her exercise regime while she was on the ward. I explained earlier that after each meal, the anorexics would have to lie on the beds for an hour, in order that the food was absorbed and not worked off or flushed down the toilet. Of course, outside the hospital there was no such curtailment. Exercise would burn off any food consumed, or be purged by laxatives or induced vomiting.

A few years later, I got the message that Angie had died. There comes a time where the body just can't take the abuse any longer. Angie was a lovely girl, but had suffered a very unhappy life.

There was a similar case with a girl called Helen, who had been an inmate before I had arrived. She was put through the program, got to her prescribed weight and was discharged. The trouble was that the doctors hadn't addressed the underlying cause of her anorexia. Therefore, three months later, paramedics brought her back in on a stretcher.

Helen was training to be a nurse at one of the teaching hospitals in London. She was a lovely girl like Angie, and had long blonde hair, but came in looking like a skeleton. She was in a bad way, her organs were packing up and she had kidney failure. She was another member of the revolving door club.

Months later, when I was visiting the Maudsley as an outpatient, I saw Helen once again. She was as thin as ever, and she told me that she could no longer eat solids but relied on liquid meals to keep her going. This was the third time that she had been admitted for her problem. I lost touch with Helen after that, so I don't know what happened to her. I hope she is all right.

I was fed up with trying to sleep in the alcove with the light on all night, so I asked to be moved. They promptly moved me to another alcove just off the men's dorm. This alcove was filthy and airless and stank, as it was right next to the men's toilet. I only stayed there one night, as I couldn't stand it. There was only one other place left for me to go on the ward, and that was in a converted linen cupboard. This room, which was at the far side of the anorexics dorm, had two iron beds and two lockers. My bed was up against the window, so it was easy for me to look out and see the Salvation Army Cross opposite.

My first roommate in the linen cupboard was a black woman called Dorothy. She was a depressive, and the main way that depression manifested itself was that she wouldn't wash. That was the first time that I observed that whereas when white people don't wash they go black, when a black person doesn't wash, they go white. Dorothy was white with dirt. Her hair was matted together, she stunk of urine and faeces, her clothes were hanging in filth and she had head lice and fleas.

Although the linen cupboard had a window in it, it wouldn't open. Therefore, it was airless and so there was no way to get rid of the pungent odour that was emitting from Dorothy. To make matters worse, for most of the day the door had to be kept closed, as it led onto the anorexics dorm. They gave me a bed in the linen cupboard on the understanding that I wouldn't be in there during the day. So to get around this, I used to hide behind the locker when the nurses checked the room, so that I could stay there and not have to spend all my time in the day room.

My friend Dana had given me a walkman, and I used to while away the hours listening to radio 4 and The Archers. I came to love radio 4; I felt it was my salvation in a world of torment. It was more of a salvation to me than the Salvation Army across the road. I still love radio 4 to this day, and never miss an episode of The Archers.

I would go down to the dining room and squirrel away some bread and jam to eat in the linen cupboard while I listened to the radio. I couldn't go down and eat a meal in the dining room because by the time I had finished, the anorexics would be back in the dorm and I would be locked out. I also used to buy myself some food on my shopping expeditions in Camberwell. Because Dorothy wasn't there during the day smelling the place out, that was my favourite time. Surrounded by misery, that safe haven made all the difference.

I went to the nurses as I could no longer stand the stench of Dorothy and I was worried that I would catch something from her. I had a very sympathetic reply. They said, 'You're no better than anyone else. You have your problems and Dorothy has hers. Dorothy's in here because she has a problem washing. Everyone in here has got their own problems, so you'll just have to learn to live with it.'

I said, 'Well, can't you make Dorothy have a bath?'

'No,' she said, 'we can't make Dorothy do anything she doesn't want to do. That's an infringement of her civil liberties'.

So I had to go on living with the stink and the fleas. I was stuck with Dorothy and her wildlife collection for about six weeks.

I regularly phoned home to speak to Mum. I could always talk to my mum, as we are on the same wavelength. However, try as I might, I could never convey the amount of suffering and misery that I was going through in hospital. It was like trying to explain colours to a blind man. Quite often, I would use a phone box at the back of the Maudsley rather than the one on the ward, for a bit of privacy. It was quite ironical that the phone box was outside a junior school. I would look through the glass of the phone box and watch the children playing. It reminded me of my schooldays, enjoyable in the early years, horrendous in the latter years. It also hit home that a lifetime ago I was going to be a teacher. That was the dream I had. I wasn't living a dream now though; I was living a nightmare. That person who was going to help children to realise their dreams and ambitions, was gone. Far from being a teacher, I was now an inmate in a mental hospital, looking at a school playground from afar. All I could do was to look through the glass of the phone box and reflect on what might have been.

After the nurse told me that there was nothing they could do about Dorothy, and that I just had to get on with it, I rang home in desperation. I was terrified of catching her nits or something worse, and I just wanted to go home. Mum told me that they were all going to Aunty Hilda's for the day, (it was a Sunday), and so I phoned her there. Aunty Hilda picked up the phone and I asked to speak to Mum, but Dad came on instead. The first thing he said to me was, 'We've just come to Hilda's for a break. Can't you let us have one day off? We're all desperate for a bit of relief from you'.

I couldn't believe what I was hearing. I know I phoned home a lot, but that was the only lifeline that I had. I was very distressed and in between sobs, I tried to explain what a living hell I was going through in the Maudsley. I tried to explain the filthy conditions that I had to live in. I tried to explain how cruel and sadistic the staff were. I tried to explain how frightened I was of some of the inmates. I told him that I just wasn't getting better there, and that I wanted to come home.

He said, 'Well, you would say that wouldn't you? You're mentally ill. You're in hospital to get better, and you're going to stay there until you are. Don't forget', he went on, 'I've got the keys to your flat, and I won't let you have them back. And I won't let you live at home either. So if you discharge yourself you'll have nowhere to go. If you go against me I'll cut you off!'

I came off the phone in tears. I couldn't believe what I had heard. I knew that Dad would do as he said and cut all ties with me if I went against him. I couldn't afford for that to happen. I needed the life support system of my family. Consequently, I was in a difficult situation. As much as I hated the nightmare of life in the Maudsley, I had no choice but to stay, as I had nowhere else to go.

Eventually they made Dorothy have a bath. After she was clean, they deemed her cured and so they let her back out into the community. In my opinion, she was no better than when she first came on the ward. Mind you, I wasn't going to argue with the decision. At last, I could sleep at night without a peg on my nose. Famous last words. My next roommate was a middle-aged lady, whose name I can't remember, who was in a wheelchair. She had also just had a colostomy. She was being treated for depression, which is hardly surprising when you're confined to a wheelchair with a colostomy bag attached to you.

They put her in the linen cupboard room because she absolutely reeked and they wanted her as far from everyone as possible. She was different from Dorothy in that she kept herself clean as far as was possible, but the trouble was that the colostomy bag wasn't changed very often. That was down to the lazy nurses and orderlies. You can imagine, as the bag filled up, the stench of waste matter became worse and worse. Even when the bag was changed, the old bag, which was full of poo, would reside in the bin until someone decided to take it away. The anorexics on the dorm would come up to me and ask me not to leave the door of the linen cupboard open, as the smell was so disgusting. It was probably putting them off their food.

I went to the staff to see if I could move somewhere else, but they refused. They said that I had tried everywhere and there was nowhere else to go. I would just have to live with it. So live with it I did, for about four weeks. It's lucky I still have a sense of humour. It's even luckier that I still have a sense of smell.

My third roommate wasn't much better than the first two. Mary was Scottish and an alcoholic. Every so often, she would come into the hospital to try to get off the drink. Mary led a very tempestuous life with a number of disreputable men. She had one of those lived in faces, which meant she looked about seventy, but was in fact only about fifty. Mary was scrupulously clean, which was a result compared to the other two, but you had to be very careful how you handled her as she could lose control as easy as could be. She also used to hallucinate. One night I was the subject of her delusion. By now, I was on quite strong drugs for my depression, therefore when I slept I was dead to the world. This particular night, I very nearly was.

I woke with a start, to find Mary on top of me holding a knife to my throat. I thought I was going to die. It was a miracle that just at that time one of the ward orderlies was doing a lethargic stroll around the ward shining her torch around the alcoves and caverns. I let out a piercing scream, and then the next thing I knew was that the orderly was pulling Mary off me. They wouldn't put Mary anywhere else, so I had to live in fear in that room every night, wondering if her hallucinations would go a step further and I would have my throat cut.

Another person I shared the linen cupboard with was a girl called Rachel. Dad and I initially noticed Rachel on my first day, when I first arrived onto the ward. She was standing by her bed space playing the flute beautifully. Rachel was an identical twin, and both she and her sister had won scholarships to Oxford. As she was about to embark upon her exciting journey of learning and knowledge, mental illness struck, as it often does at that age. Rachel was diagnosed with manic depression. It was quite sad as her sister went on to Oxford and Rachel went to the Maudsley.

Like many manic-depressives, Rachel was highly intelligent, although prone to highs and lows in mood and behaviour. She was also very promiscuous and if she got a chance to leave the hospital she would spend her evening sleeping with anyone she could find.

There was an elderly man on the ward who was at one time a graphic artist on The Beatles album covers. He had fallen upon hard times, became an alcoholic and ended up in the Maudsley. He was rather seedy, old and drink sodden, but even so, the rumour was that Rachel had slept with him. When she shared the linen cupboard with me, she would be missing some nights and come in at two or three in the morning, having carried on in a rampant way with anyone she could find. The staff were always annoyed at her, probably because it meant having to wake up to let her in.

My last roommate was a girl called Yvonne. She had similar problems to me, in that she also was unable to cope, had depression and an eating disorder. Yvonne lived in a bed-sit, and after she was admitted to the Maudsley, her landlady decided that she didn't want anyone with mental health problems living in her flat. So she packed all Yvonne's things into black bin bags and left them out on the street. A friend of Yvonne's collected the stuff for her, but it meant that not only was she an inmate in a mental hospital, she was also homeless.

When the depression got the better of me, I would find a quiet corner and cry. When Yvonne got depressed and angry, she would smash windows. Yvonne was the girl that the useless trainee Spanish doctor confused with me. I kept in contact with Yvonne after she left the Maudsley, and she did eventually get a flat nearby, in one of those awful soulless tower block places. I went to visit her once whilst I was en route to the Maudsley as an outpatient. She was struggling to cope in this flat, which was very basic. It was one of those places that would give anyone depression. I think Yvonne joined the revolving door club, in that she would be in and out of hospital for the rest of her life. I corresponded with her for a few years, but then I stopped getting replies, so I don't know what became of her.

What added to the general filth of the ward was the fact that there was only one cleaner, who was also quite old and extremely lazy. She was also an alcoholic. She used to hide in the broom cupboard and drink. She used to stink of drink and by the end of the day she could hardly walk or string two sentences together. When you consider that the standards of hygiene of many of the patients on the ward left a lot to be desired, having a cleaner like that was not a very good idea.

There was a filth-encrusted kitchen on the ward, which, several times during the day, the staff opened up to allow patients to use. You could go in there and make yourself a cup of coffee and a piece of toast. The cleaner never went near it, which was evident from the state of the place. The surfaces were ingrained with grime, and the cups and plates were disgusting. Everything needed sterilising before you could use them. We would tell each other if there were a few slices of bread available and make teas and coffees for one another.

Just those simple acts of having a cup of tea and a slice of toast in a filthy kitchen, with people who you knew were going through the same struggles as you, was like a refuge. I almost said that it was an asylum, which of course it was. We would do the best for each other with what little we had. Again, it reminded me of prisoner of war films, and the comradeship in adversity.

One of the male patients had at one time been an eminent professor of theology at one of the major London universities, and was in the Maudsley after suffering a massive breakdown. One of the things I remember about him was that he used to walk up and down the ward spouting inconsequential and odd bits of scripture, in a manic way.

When we used to go down to breakfast in the morning, he would get about five boiled eggs and erect them into a sort of pyramid shape. He would then sit and stare at these eggs, as if they were the most amazing conundrum, and have no idea what to do with them. None of the nurses ever came over to help him to remove the shells so that he could eat them. This went on day after day. He would collect his eggs, sit and look at them, and then be led back to the ward without having any breakfast.

Another thing about this man was that he wouldn't wash. He was so filthy that one day the orderlies made him take a bath, (so it seems that they could if they wanted to). As there were no baths on the male dorm, the male patients used to use our baths. After he had his bath and returned to his dorm, the orderlies came up to me and told me that it was my turn to have a bath. I had told them that I had trouble coping in the flat including having a bath, so they decided that they were going to observe me having a bath to try to help me cope.

I got ready to have this bath, but when I looked in it, it was absolutely disgusting. The only vacant bath was the one that the theology professor had just vacated. The accumulation of weeks of dirt and scum from this man was caked on the sides. They expected me to get in it after him. I would have got out dirtier than when I got in. It was a health hazard. There were pubic hairs clinging to the sides of this grime-blackened bath. I could have collected them together and made a Brillo pad out of them. I went to try to find the alcoholic cleaner to see if she would clean it, but she had locked herself in the broom cupboard with a bottle of scotch, so no one would see her for the rest of the day.

A nurse came up to me and said, 'Now you mustn't be obsessive about it. Just get in it and get on with it'.

I did find some Vim or something and a cloth and tried to scrape off some of the worst of the filth before I got in it. I felt sick with the thought of having to lie in this revolting bath, but I had no choice. I can tell you, it did no good towards helping me with my problem.

Another brilliant whim from the medical staff to help me with my cleaning problems was to put me with the elderly, lazy, alcoholic cleaner to help her. What an inspired decision that was. To put someone that has cleaning difficulties with a raging alcoholic that did no cleaning. They told me it was to help me. I personally think that they wanted someone to clean the ward, and not someone that hid in cupboards getting drunk. She gave me all the disgusting and filthy jobs that she didn't want to do, not that she did anything herself. I more or less had to get on with it myself. Even if you were capable, fit, and healthy and didn't mind cleaning, you would be fighting a losing battle here. For example, underneath the beds were clusters of fluff that were so large it was as if someone had just sheared a sheep in there.

I did a bit of hoovering and dusting, especially around my room. I reasoned that if I had to clean, I might as well clean where I slept. Not that it really made much difference. Most of my roommates would hardly have made it to Vogue magazine. I drew the line at cleaning the toilets. I have described what the baths were like, (they were all like the one I tried to clean), but you will have to use your imagination as to how the toilets looked. Repulsive is too mild a word. Therefore, I concentrated my efforts on polishing the coffee tables. These were as hideous as the rest of the ward, with ingrained tea and coffee stains, and other stains that I wouldn't like to study too hard, but it was the least nauseating job I could do.

There are no prizes for guessing that this 'therapy' did my phobia no good. If anything, it put me back. The fact that I was dealing with filth everyday, and worse still it was not even my filth, made it even worse. Top marks to the Maudsley for Psychotherapy.

Years later, I was walking past Westminster Cathedral in Victoria. Most of the shops had shut and I happened to look in one of the shop doorways to see a figure wrapped in old sacking. I did a double take because I thought that I recognized the face. It was the professor of theology. I know that he had a family, as they had visited him in hospital, and someone had told me that he had a large house. I can only assume that his family wanted nothing to do with him now. I thought it was sad that a man with a brilliant mind could come to this. It just goes to show that none of us is safe from mental illness. It can strike anyone at any time and the stigma that goes with it blights your life. Going from being a professor in a top university to living in a shop doorway is a sad journey, and one that I wouldn't wish on my worst enemy.

It is an unfortunate fact that suicide is a by-product of life on a mental ward. I saw many people die while I was in the Maudsley. There was an attractive woman called Melanie, a manic-depressive, who was on my ward. She had been married three times and had three children. She was very attractive with long, golden hair and beautiful eyes. Like Rachel, when Melanie was on a 'high', she got very promiscuous. She got friendly with one of the male patients, an alcoholic Scotsman. This man also suffered from depression, and his illness was getting worse. One day his illness got the better of him and he slashed his wrists. The staff called the paramedics out from Kings Hospital opposite, but unfortunately, on this occasion, they were too late and the man died.

Later on, I was on my way to the toilet and heard some moaning noises coming from the cubicle next to me. I tapped on the closed door and asked if everything was all right, but got no response. When I looked down, I noticed blood seeping under the door. I rushed to get some help, and a couple of the nurses quickly came and managed to get the door open. It was Melanie. She had slashed her wrists in despair of her friend dying. Once again, the paramedics were called in and they took her to the accident and emergency department of King's hospital. Rapid action from all involved had prevented a potential suicide on that occasion, but it was lucky that I happened to be in the right place at the right time to get help.

The only postscript that I can add to this story is that about two years later, I went back to the Maudsley as an outpatient, and I saw Melanie on the ward. I can only hope she never tried to repeat her action.

There was another very sad case of a little man, who reminded me of a leprechaun. He wasn't Irish, but he was tiny with a long beard and long, straggly hair. He suffered from depression and stayed on the general ward. As the staff allowed him to go out of the ward, he would run errands for those who were not. Consequently, he would toddle off to Camberwell to pick up the daily order of tobacco or coffee. The shops were closed on Sundays, so he would go over to King's hospital and use their shop.

One Sunday this man had taken an overdose of drugs, which he had been saving up and never told anyone what he had done. Meanwhile one of the other patients, (the Beatles graphic designer), had asked him to get some tobacco. As it was a Sunday he duly went off to King's hospital shop, and brought back the tobacco. He handed it over, collapsed, and died. The staff and paramedics tried in vain to save him, but it was too late. I found it ironical that this poor man, who was obviously at the end of his tether, still found time to run an errand even while the drugs were poisoning his body.

I came across a number of nice, selfless people during my six months as an inpatient; people whose only crime was to have a mental illness.

There was another nice man on the ward, whose name was Keith, who suffered from schizophrenia. Keith was in his thirties and was married with two teenage girls. His wife and girls visited him on a few occasions, but then his wife decided that she had had enough. She could no longer cope with his psychological problems. Therefore, while he was in the Maudsley, she started proceedings for a divorce. He was now homeless, so the Maudsley found him a place to stay. It was in a bed-sit in a run down house. By all accounts, it was a depressing place, as they usually are.

After Keith moved in, the hospital gave him an appointment for the outpatients' clinic a fortnight later. He never turned up. The police were asked to go round to see if everything was all right. On getting no reply at the door, they broke into Keith's flat to find him hanging from the light flex. He had been there some time.

There was a man on the ward, whose name I can't recall, who had a girlfriend and together they had a baby. However, the girlfriend didn't want anything to do with this man, and stopped him from seeing his child. It really broke this man's heart that he couldn't see his son, and he would sit on his bed and sob. Nevertheless, if he saw someone else who was upset or distressed, he would play his guitar for them. He was so selfless that he put his own problems to one side to try to help others. Sometimes of an evening, he would sit in one of the interview rooms and play his guitar and some of us would sit and listen to him.

He attempted several times to get back with his girlfriend, but she just didn't want to know. This made him more and more depressed to the point where he could go on no longer. He killed himself by slashing his wrists. I watched the ambulance men carry this lovely, gentle man, off the ward with a blanket over his face.

I find it hard to do justice to the tragic and heartbreaking circumstances of these people. Over a period of six months, I built up a rapport with many of the patients. We had a comradeship that is hard to explain to anyone who has not been in similar circumstances. We all looked out for each other, would help each other, and rally round if someone was in a particularly bad way. Therefore, if someone killed himself or herself, it hit you as if they were a life long friend. People become very close to each other in an organization that takes away all your creature comforts and even all your dignity. I would imagine a similar thing happened to prisoners of war. These human beings, (because that's what they were, not a collection of illnesses,) became my friends. Some of them were very sick, and were in hospital through no fault of their own, but many of them were nice, unassuming human beings and they were kind to me. That is more than I can say about the majority of the medical staff.

After a while when you see people being readmitted a couple of months after being discharged, you realize that more often than not, there is no cure; there is no quick fix. If you had a broken leg, you would go to a general hospital, where the doctors would fix it before sending you home again. That doesn't happen with mental illnesses.

One day, when this awareness hit me particularly forcefully, I asked a coloured nurse, with tears in my eyes, 'Is there any hope for me? Will I get better and leave this place and not come back?' With typical insight and compassion that most of the nurses on the ward had, she answered, 'You'll be like all the others. Your case is classic. You'll be part of the revolving door syndrome. You'll be in and out for the rest of your life.'

Even as ill and drugged as I was at the time, I thought how stupid and unfeeling it was for her to say that. Even if that were the case, it was a very unwise thing to say. That statement may be enough to push someone over the edge and end it all. However, I'm quite stubborn, (Dad says it comes from my red hair). I refused to give in. That tactless statement from that nurse, gave me the impetus and determination to say to myself, 'I am never coming back to a place like this again. They can't solve my problems for me, so once I get out, I'm never coming back.'

Not all the nursing staff were complete sods though. There was one student nurse, who had transferred from general nursing, called Hilary. She was excellent. She tried to help me and listened to me, and I felt that she was someone that I could relate to. The only trouble was, all the patients wanted to speak to her, as she was the only one who seemed to care. Therefore, I only managed about ten minutes twice a week with her. Nevertheless, those ten minutes made all the difference, as she made me feel like a human being again. If only all the staff were like her, my stay would have been a bit more bearable. My only concern is that the rest of the staff did not corrupt her, turning her like them.

One other decent night nurse started towards the end of my stay. She was very pleasant and kind, but she wasn't particularly able in any other way, as she wasn't as medically proficient as Hilary was. Nevertheless, she wouldn't make us hurry at the washbasins, or shout at us to get to bed because she was going to turn the lights out so that she could get her head down. These two were really the only members of staff that I received any kindness or compassion or understanding from, in all the time I was there.

Occasionally a trainee psychiatrist would come over from the teaching part of the hospital to see me. They would come to interview 'exhibit A', as that is what it felt like. They would ask all sorts of questions pertaining to their particular field of research, but you felt that they were only working on their next essay.

I went to another part of the Maudsley to have a brain scan. This was to see if there was anything organically wrong with me. There wasn't. A psychologist also gave me a test to see what my intelligence levels were like. She told me that in some areas, for example verbal skills and comprehension, I was above average intelligence. In other areas, maths and puzzle solving, I was below average intelligence. This was somewhat of a conundrum for them, as they couldn't work out why for some things I didn't have a normal capacity, whereas in others I had way above normal capacity. I didn't want to confuse them more by telling them that when I read a map, I have to turn it around to face the direction I'm travelling.

After being in the Maudsley for a fortnight, the doctors called me to a meeting to discuss my case. These meetings took place on Wednesday afternoons, and to get to them you had to go through a fire door near the anorexic dorm and down the fire escape to the yard below. There was a Portacabin in the yard, which was the consulting room. The doctor asked me some perfunctory questions about how I was, and then told me that he was going to put me on a drug called Imipramine, which was a tricyclic drug.

In those days, for general depression, doctors mainly prescribed tricyclic drugs. If they didn't work, they would put you on a drug type called M.A.O.I (monoamine oxidase inhibitors). However, they didn't like putting patients on those right away, as they had dietary restrictions associated with them, and a possibility of liver damage. There were a number of tricyclic drugs to choose from. If a patient needed sedating, doctors would prescribe Amitriptyline. This drug was no good for me, as part of my illness was that I was tired all the time. I didn't need a drug to sedate me further. Imipramine didn't give you energy, or allow you to do break dancing, (I would be on them now if they did), but they were slightly less sedating than Amitriptyline.

I stayed on that drug for about three months. Three months was the norm for getting patients settled on a drug, before being set free. Having 'served' my three months, I was going to be discharged. Unfortunately, Imipramine was making me dizzy and in fact, I had fainted on a number of occasions. I think that it lowers your blood pressure and as I already have very low blood pressure, it made things worse. I knew that I couldn't go home in that state, but the doctors ignored my views. I phoned home and told them what was happening and Dad agreed to come up to the hospital and have a word with my doctor. He argued my case with medical staff, saying that the drug was not agreeing with me, and that it wasn't safe to let me out in that condition. Fortunately, they listened to him and decided to keep me in for a bit longer while they tried me on another drug.

They put me on Desipramine to see how I fared on that. That drug had a slightly better effect on me as I didn't get the dizziness on it. On the negative side, I had to stay in hospital longer than

I should have if the first drug had worked. I was very grateful to my dad for coming up that day to argue my case. As much as I hated being in the Maudsley, there was no way that I could have coped the way I was.

One of the anorexic patients from the eating disorder section was a six foot two, blond, blue eyed, very attractive man with a lovely smile and a gentle nature. His name was Karl. It was, and still is, quite uncommon for a male to be anorexic, as it is predominantly a female illness.

All the female patients flocked round Karl, like bees round a honey pot. Being shy, and because of my experiences in the past, I kept my distance. I admired him from afar, because I felt that nobody would want to be associated with me. By the time I arrived on the ward, Karl had been there for some time and had gone through the fattening up process. His target weight was about thirteen stone, and the first time I saw him he was about eleven stone. Therefore, I had never really seen him exceptionally thin.

Karl was completely charming to everyone he met, although he had many problems underneath, which he tried to conceal. As he was coming to the end of his treatment period, he spent more and more time in the day room area. The system for the anorexics was that, as they put on weight and ate relatively normally in the anorexic dining area, the staff allowed them to have their snacks in the day room, away from supervision. As time went on, they could have their main meals alone, before going home for weekends, prior to being discharged.

One day I saw him sitting in the alcove of the day room, away from the main day room area, where he usually sat. There was a coffee table and half a dozen plastic chairs, and he was sitting with Yasmin, Clare, and some of the girls from the anorexic dorm. I was sitting in a corner by myself, because I knew better than to try to mix with any group. He saw me sitting by myself, and called over to me, 'Sue, come on over and join us'. That meant so much to me, as I had always felt rejected, especially from the in crowd. From then on, he would always include me in that little group that sat around the coffee table in the alcove.

Karl seemed to be unaware of the affect that he had on the crowd he had around him, especially the girls. That was obviously due to his lack of self worth and his emotional problems. He had a chronic lack of self-confidence and he immersed himself with the fact that he had put on weight, and he couldn't handle that.

Not being fully aware of this at the time, I couldn't understand how someone who was so good looking, had such a lovely personality and was so nice, could be so humble and be so unaware of the effect he was creating. Karl had the ability to make you feel special. Whoever he talked to would have his undivided attention; he would make them feel important. I suppose it came with his humility, which he had in abundance.

One day Karl asked me to buy him a jar of coffee when I went to the shops. When I brought it back I was frightened, because instead of sitting with a group of girls, today he sat alone. I was shy and felt inadequate and unworthy to talk to him on my own. He saw me standing there, smiled, and beckoned me over. He was so grateful to me for buying him the coffee, and he made such a big thing of it, that I came away really feeling good about myself.

Something that I heard about, although it was before my time in the Maudsley, was that Rachel, (the flute-playing identical twin), had asked him to marry her. It was mainly Rachel's idea, and Karl would go along with anything, as I later found out. Karl asked his mother and father if they would buy an engagement ring for them. This engagement had an added significance for Karl, as his mother and father had also met in a mental hospital. Karl and Rachel, in their respective illnesses, felt that history was going to repeat itself. They thought that if they were together, then everything would be all right and all their problems would be solved.

However, the engagement didn't last very long. From what I can gather, Rachel decided that it wasn't going to work and so called off the engagement. Karl always went along with what anyone wanted just to keep the peace. His self-obsession with what he ate took precedence over every conscious thought.

Karl went home one weekend, and when he came back, he was very distressed. He said that the weekend hadn't gone well, and that he spent most of it in his room. He said that he was unable to have a meal with his family. In fact, he was unable to keep up with any of the eating plans of the hospital. Karl's parents came up to speak to the staff about him still being ill. However, as far as Professor Russell's plan went Karl had spent his requisite three months on the ward, was up to the required weight, and therefore he was ready to go home. He went soon after.

About six weeks later, I was doing my usual constitution around Ruskin Park, (having evaded the searchlights and the dogs to avoid nail packing duty), when I saw a lone figure sitting on a park bench. He was wearing a tartan lumber jacket, and looked gaunt, thin, and ill. I had to do a double take as I thought that I recognised him. When I got up closer I realised to my dismay that it was Karl. He had lost about two stone and had shaved most of his long blond hair off.

I went over to speak to him and once again, he made me feel like I was the one person in the world that he wanted to talk to. He wouldn't talk about his weight loss. In common with most anorexics, it's a taboo subject. I said goodbye as he left for his outpatient's appointment, not thinking that I would ever see him again.

After serving my six months in the Maudsley, the parole board- I mean medical panel, told me that I was about to be released. I was on Desipramine, which was helping, although I was still unable to cope in the flat. Having said that, I was less anxious and less depressed now, so they decided to let me out into the community, just as I was starting to have fun. I went back to the ward, packed my few possessions in my bag, and finally left the Maudsley on the 26th January 1989.

In summing up my stay, I have to say that the Maudsley did help in getting me on Desipramine, which helped with my depression. Desipramine helped me for about eighteen months, after which time it was no longer effective. Apart from that, I certainly didn't get any help as far as coping on my own in the flat, or coming to terms with or dealing with the myriad of problems that I was suffering from.

I have concluded that the mental hospital cannot cure you. It can treat your symptoms, but it just hasn't time to psychoanalyse every sane patient and get to the cause of their symptoms; even if it does, it can only diagnose the cause, not get down to doing something about it. If a person is depressed because he or she is shy and lonely, for instance, doctors can't provide him or her with the companionship they need. Most mentally ill people need a lot of understanding and support. People will sympathise with a broken leg, but not with fits of crying and unhappiness. 'Pull yourself together' is a well worn phrase from individuals who don't understand. If only it were that simple.

Sometimes people with a psychological illness have to go into a mental hospital. When - or if - they come out, society labels them neurotic. Even seemingly intelligent people, who should know better, frequently treat them with contempt. Like racial discrimination, it's all based on ignorance and fear. Even if you can understand people outside of the health profession acting in an ignorant way, due to fear or not understanding, what is the excuse for those working in mental institutions? What do they have to fear?

At the end of the day, we are all human beings with human frailties. Any one of us can develop a mental illness, the same as any one of us can get cancer or heart disease. Therefore, everyone deserves to be treated like a human being. Just because an illness is invisible, unlike a broken leg for example, doesn't make it is any less valid. It also doesn't make it any less painful.

Looking back, my time in the Maudsley was one of the worst periods of my life. On the plus side, I did meet some wonderful people in there, who had tremendous crosses to bear, and I was part of a brilliant solidarity that stemmed from the adverse conditions in which we all had to survive. However, overall, if I had my time over again I would never have gone in. It didn't solve any of my problems; in fact, I think it exacerbated them to a degree. It certainly opened my eyes to another side of life, and I will never forget the anguish and suffering that people, who became my friends, went through.

LIFE ON THE OUTSIDE

'Free at last, free at last'. That was the dream of Martin Luther King. However, what is freedom? I was out of the hellhole called the Maudsley that I had inhabited for six months, but of course, I wasn't free. I was still a prisoner of my illness. I would never be free until I was free from my illness.

I sat in the armchair at Mum and Dad's house, and felt petrified. How would I cope in my flat? Although Desipramine helped a bit, I still had depression, I still couldn't cope with living on my own and my eating problem was as bad as ever. Dad asked me if I wanted to stay the night. However, I told him no, I had to go. I had to face the fear. If I put it off, it would be harder for me in the long run. So, Dad took me home and I walked into my cold, lonely flat.

Even today, I still have bad dreams about being alone in Martins Court, of being unable to face the hoovering or the dusting, in fact any other normal household chores. I was trapped in a downward spiral of extreme anxiety. The more I tried to cope, the more anxious I became, which meant I was less able to cope. The walls seemed to be closing in on me, making me want to run away. However, there was nowhere for me to go. I couldn't even go out, as I was frightened of people and there were some very undesirable types in Martins Court. In every sense, I was trapped.

Because I couldn't cope with washing up, I would eat off paper plates and drink out of plastic cups. Mum did all my washing and ironing so that I didn't have to do that. I didn't make a mess;

therefore, I didn't have to clean up afterwards. It was all coping strategies, really.

My life in the flat became quite insular. It consisted of trying and failing to do housework. Everything was a major effort. For example, if I were to have a bath and wash my hair, it would take me all day; not because I was fastidious nor had OCD, but because of the effort involved. I had extreme fatigue, and the anxiety of gearing up to having a bath and then clearing up afterwards exacerbated that. My stay in the Maudsley had done nothing to reduce my phobias and fears. I got very frustrated and hated myself for not being able to do those simple everyday tasks. That frustration led to massive binges. I ate so much that I could not stand up, my stomach was bloated and in pain, and I would have to go to bed to sleep it off, much as an alcoholic would sleep off a drinking binge.

The next morning I would wake up, feel disgusted with myself, and hate myself even more for what I had done. This led to a terrible black depression, which meant I could do nothing; and so it went on, day after day. In order to try to help my situation, I was still an outpatient at the Maudsley. Now that I was no longer an inpatient, I told them of my eating disorder, and so the eating disorder specialists saw me too. The hospital also organised a family meeting. The idea was that a psychologist would interview my family and me while other specialists watched us behind a two-way mirror. They wanted to find out the reasons behind my psychological problems. Again, the family closed ranks and they would give nothing away about our home life. They kept everything hidden away. Consequently, it was a waste of time.

Nothing really helped or worked for me. The outpatient part of the Maudsley was as dire as the in-patient part. It was just as soul destroying and just as dirty. The receptionists were anything but welcoming and gave short shrift to everyone. Many desperate people there were in a worse state than I was. One man came in with a pit bull terrier and two rottweillers, and he was threatening to set them on people if he didn't get any help. I was very frightened, but I remember thinking, 'What else can you do if this is the end of the line for you, and there's nowhere else to go?'

Every time I went, a different doctor saw me. They were all trainees, and each one said, 'Well, if you tell me your name and what your problems are, I'll try to help you'. As a result, each time I went I would have to start again from scratch, while they filled in a form. At the end, they would all tell me to keep taking the medication, and away I would go until the next time.

I came home after a visit to outpatients, sat on the stairs of Martins Court, and cried for about 5 hours. I knew there were no answers. I was so desperate at the time, that if I'd had the courage, I would have taken an overdose and ended it all. I knew that I was wasting my time going to the Maudsley outpatients. Why did I keep going, you may well ask. You see, I looked upon my trips to the Maudsley as an outing. It gave me a purpose in life. I had little else. I would combine my visit to the hospital with a walk round Ruskin Park, which

I loved, and a trip to Camberwell to look round the shops.

I walked a lot in those days, in fact I still like walking now, but during my time in Martins Court I walked to keep me out of the flat. In the mornings, I would do what I could in the flat and work towards my reward in the afternoon, which was a walk. I loved walking down all the country lanes, through the parks, and by the river. Not only did the fresh air and beautiful scenery do wonders for my state of mind, it also had an added bonus of not being near any of my old haunts that I tried to avoid. If I had to go into town for shopping, I would use all the back doubles and thus avoid meeting people or passing places that had bad memories for me, like the Blue Arrow building.

I was trying to make the best of the shipwreck that was my life. I still lived for Radio 4 and The Archers, and had it on whenever I was in. Mum and Dad persuaded me to buy a portable black and white television, but I could never settle to watch it on my own. Even today, if I'm on my own, I much prefer listening to the radio.

Looking back with hindsight, I was terribly unhappy, my anxiety was through the roof, and my depression was black. I wasn't coping or holding together at all. Even though my family supported me a lot, I don't think that I should have been trying to cope in a flat on my own.

I used to go to Mum and Dad's every Sunday for lunch. To spare them and me any humiliation, they used to drive me into the garage and I would go into the house through the back door. That way no neighbours would see me, or if they did, they would have no opportunity to question me about my life. I was an embarrassment to my family. They were so proud of me when I got the top A levels in my school, then went on to teachers training college. I was nothing to be proud of now. I had failed at everything I had tried to do. If I managed to have a bath and wash my hair, then that was a major achievement for me.

I didn't go to any family gatherings and events. My family thought it best if I was kept out of sight and therefore out of mind. I didn't go to any weddings, christenings or funerals, and so no relative ever saw me, apart from Aunty Norah, Uncle Bert and Aunty Hilda, who occasionally came over for tea on a Sunday. If anyone asked about me, Mum would say, 'Oh, she's doing fine, living in her own flat'. Then quickly change the subject. For many of my relatives, it must have seemed that I had died.

Even on Boxing Day, when Mum and Dad would go to Bert and Norah's, I would stay at home in my flat. I had no inclination of going, as I felt so ill all the time, and I certainly was not in a festive mood. Apart from that, I didn't want to be in the car while Mum and Dad had a row over which direction they should go in. Dad was a terrible navigator, but he always knew best. So they got to Mill Hill, (where Bert and Norah lived), via John O' Groats. On those occasions, Julie would stay with me. By this time, Julie had a car of her own, and so was more independent. Although she was not a very confidant driver, she could get to my flat all right. I used to enjoy the times we spent together. She would come down every Friday, (for Friday

Folk), although she would quite often go home Friday evening and then come back the next day and spend Saturday evening and Sunday morning with me. Sundays we would go to the Mass centre, and then Julie would drive us to Mum and Dad's for lunch, via the garage.

While Julie was with me, I had more of a normal life. I didn't binge eat as much, and I was able to cope slightly better, albeit in a limited way. Having said all that, by this time Julie was getting sick herself. She wasn't coping with her job in the civil Service; therefore, she was beginning to get some of the problems that were to develop later on. Consequently, some of our time together was spent going over her life and problems while I would counsel her, so they were not all happy times. Nevertheless, in the midst of our unhappy lives, my flat was a haven for us both.

By this time, my confidence had gone completely concerning working. My illness was such that I couldn't cope with anything. However, I did want to contribute to society and do something constructive. With Mum's encouragement, I decided that I would do some voluntary work. She saw an advert in the local paper for volunteers at St. Raphael's home for the blind. I phoned the home to see if they needed anyone to read to the guests, as I had a good speaking voice. The woman that ran the home, a Mrs. Colfer, invited me along for an interview.

I knew Mrs. Colfer, as two of her children went to my school. Consequently, she also knew me. At least, she knew the girl I once was. That is, the girl who won the Canon Keanan cup and the girl who got the top A level grades. When she found out that I wanted to be a volunteer in her home, she couldn't believe her luck. She thought that she was getting the high flyer that I once was. Obviously, she didn't know my history since those days, and I was in no hurry to tell her.

Every Wednesday afternoon in the communal lounge, there was a book club. One of my jobs was to read to these ladies from a book chosen by them. I didn't have much of an audience for those readings. Out of 26 guests about five came. That's because not all the residents were totally blind and they could read for themselves or else they could read Braille. The ones that did come seemed to be the most cantankerous of the lot. One old lady always fell asleep and snored heavily during the readings. I can only hope that it was due to old age, and not a criticism of me. Two other old ladies didn't hide the fact that they were critics. They would pick me up on everything I said and did. Yet another was in the final stages of dementia, so I could have been reading her the phone book for all she knew. Apart from that, they were all very old and very frail. About once a month one of them would die. (Not of boredom, I hasten to add.)

The membership was never replaced when one of them dropped off the twig. As a result, my audience got smaller and smaller, until after about four months it was just the lady with dementia, me and the phone book.

I would have given up apart from one person, Dorothy. When I first met Dorothy, I knew that we were going to get along. For a start, I considered it a good omen that we shared the same surname, Kennedy. Dorothy was 82 when I met her and a wonderful person.

She had not had an easy life, as she had been totally blind from the age of two. She lived at home with her mother and father. When her mother died, her father tried to cope for both of them. Her father was bombastic and a bully and had not been easy to live with. He couldn't cope with looking after them both and eventually Dorothy's sister and her husband took them both in.

During the early part of the 20th century, if you had a disability, society treated you like a second-class citizen. Things have improved since then, although not nearly enough. Dorothy spent her day sitting in her room, making raffia baskets, which she sold to help pay for her keep.

Dorothy had a sad life, and lived on the periphery of things. She was never allowed an opinion, was always talked over, and was only brought out of her room for meals, after which she had to return. She told of her despondency of schools for the blind, which were privately run ventures by people who neither knew nor cared how to look after the students. In her school, the other students bullied her and the headmistress was a tyrant.

After her father and sister died, Dorothy lived in various homes. She had to share a room in each of these places, and so never had any privacy. Later in life when she had found St. Raphael's, she considered herself lucky. At least she had a room to herself, where she could sit and listen to the radio in peace. She loved radio 4 and especially The Archers. We had a lot in common.

After all that life had thrown at Dorothy, you could forgive her if she was bitter and cynical. However, nothing was further from the truth. She was a wonderful person and she never lost her sense of humour. She was very bright, and although she spent her life sitting in a chair, she was aware of world events and could talk on any subject. I think that people who moan about the weather or rubbish on the telly or other trivia, should spend an hour with the likes of Dorothy, to put life into perspective.

The only other person that cared for Dorothy was her niece, the daughter of the sister she used to live with. She would come and visit Dorothy and take care of any business for her.

I visited Dorothy every Thursday afternoon for about four years. She rarely left her room, but she told me that one of the things she wished she could do was go for a walk. Consequently, every nice day I would take her round the local park or we would go for a picnic. She came to my flat on one occasion, for her birthday. I sent a taxi for her and did her a salad. I wasn't capable of doing anything else due to my illness. We sat on my balcony and chatted about everything and nothing. It was nothing special; nevertheless, you would have thought that I had given her gold. She really appreciated it, but I too really appreciated her company. We were good for each other and I had made a good friend.

As my life spiralled more and more out of control, and there were more things going on around me, I had less time to visit Dorothy. I would visit at Christmas, Easter, and occasionally during the summer school holidays, but not very often. My illness precluded that. Although it was not my fault, I never forgave myself for letting Dorothy down. Apart from her niece, I was the only person that she had.

One day, out of the blue, I got a letter from Dorothy's niece saying that she had died. She said that her funeral was in Gloucester and early in the morning. There was no way that I could get to it. She put in her letter that Dorothy had appreciated the times that I had visited her. I cried my eyes out. I was upset that I was unable to visit Dorothy during her last days and that I couldn't even get to her funeral.

So that was the end of Dorothy's life. Bless her; she went out of this world without any fanfares or hordes of mourners. She died as she had lived, alone. At least I know in my heart of hearts, that if there is a heaven, a lovely person like Dorothy will be there.

As well as my voluntary work at St. Raphael's, I also wanted to rekindle my love of literature. I had always loved literature and I wanted to regenerate what I felt I had lost, due to my illness. I found out from the library about the Workers' Education Association. These were set up at the beginning of the 20th Century for working people who hadn't had a proper education.

I signed up for a literacy class and an art appreciation class. I really loved these classes. There was no pressure, no examinations, but it was very enlightening. I highly recommend them to anyone who wants to add to their knowledge without any pressure.

As an aside, as I was leaving one of these classes I almost bumped straight into Diana, Princess of Wales. She was opening the Fleetville Community Centre. She looked gorgeous. Having read about her, I realise that she too had problems, some similar to mine. As I have said, mental illness can strike anyone.

I went to the W.E.A for a year and signed up for the next year. Unfortunately, a teacher who I knew from Nicholas Breakspear School joined. She had many questions about my life and at the time I went along with Mum and Dad's opinion of keeping things to myself, therefore I left the W.E.A. I was sad to leave as I really enjoyed it.

I tried to have a holiday every year if I could, normally with Julie and my friend Kathy. Nothing special, just a few days in cheap accommodation, as none of us had much money. We went to Oxford in1989, Westgate in '90 and Cambridge in '91. I used to organise these trips, and because we had no transport, we went everywhere by bus or train.

The first holiday in Oxford was excellent. We stayed in student accommodation, and as it was at the end of season, we got a place designed for 12 to ourselves. Mind you, it didn't get off to a very auspicious start. None of us are very good navigators. In fact, I was the best of the three of us, which begs the question as to how we got anywhere. I managed to get us all on the right train, and we arrived in Oxford. However, that was as good as I could do. We were in Oxford all right, but we had no idea how to get to our accommodation. We got on a bus and told the driver where we were staying and he dropped us as near as he could. Still not sure of the way to our digs, Kathy and I stood with all our suitcases outside a large building, while Julie wandered off to look for our accommodation. She finally found the college we were staying at, and told the woman on the reception desk that we were there. She said to her, 'You didn't come down the country lane to get here, did you?'

'Yes', said Julie.

'Oh no,' said the woman, 'we have warned all the female students here not to go that way. A girl was attacked there last night.'

Julie went white as a sheet, but luckily, she didn't have to return via the country lane. There was a short cut back to where we were. Meanwhile, back where we were waiting, people started coming out of the building carrying banners. It turns out that the building was Pergamon Press, owned by Robert Maxwell. All the printers were coming out on strike, over union recognition. We couldn't move because of all our cases, and besides, we had to stay where we were so that Julie could find us. Eventually we were surrounded by pickets waving their banners and chanting their chants. We would have joined in if we had known the words. The press turned up to cover the story and the photographers were taking photos of the strikers, plus us two. The most unlikely flying pickets you could think of. Julie came back about an hour later to find us in the middle of a major dispute. She made Kathy put down the banner reading 'One out- All out.' and we headed off for our digs, while she regaled the story to us of the attack the night before.

A few days later, after a day out, we returned to our accommodation to find all the doors open. After what Julie had told us that first day, we naturally feared the worst. Happily, it was only the cleaning staff who had left the doors open. We breathed a sigh of relief, but I went to bed at night wishing that I had a baseball bat handy. Apart from that, it was a lovely holiday.

Although I no longer went on holiday with Mum and Dad, the Westgate holiday I booked resembled one of Dad's specials. Thinking we were getting something nice but ending up in a crap hole. I had done all my research, and the flat I had booked for us was in the Tourist Information Guide. There was a photo of it and it looked lovely, and the ad said it had all mod cons. It was nearly right, but it should have read 'A complete con.' A couple called the Hanson's owned the flat, which was above their flat. The flat that they showed the tourist information guide was another one that their son used. The flat they gave us was disgusting.

Mr. Hanson was an absolute slob, complete with beer belly and string vest. He was aggressive to us from the first minute. He obviously knew he was in the wrong by letting out this dump instead of the one he advertised, so he was on the defensive from the start. He knew that he wouldn't have any trouble from us three, shy girls. We had to scrub everything before we could use them. The cups looked like something had died in the bottom of them. There was a veil of cobwebs hanging from every surface. There were no light shades, just bare bulbs hanging from the ceiling. The light switches were hanging from the walls with all their wires exposed.

I noticed a tiny portable TV in the corner and I remembered that there was also supposed to be a radio. When I asked him where the radio was he snarled at me, 'What do you think this is? What do you want for yer money?'

'What you advertised in your brochure is what we want.' I answered. 'Now give us a decent TV and radio and get this place cleaned up before I get the health inspectors down here.'

Well, that's what I thought, at least. Of course, I didn't say anything. None of us did. The bullies won again.

He showed us round the rest of the squat, as that was how it felt to me, and took us into the bathroom. He pointed to the bath, which was painted bright pink.

'I've just painted this bath,' he said, 'so don't go running any 'ot water in it. I don't want all the paint coming off.'

Chance would be a fine thing anyway. There was a meter for the hot water and we fed this thing like a fruit machine. We never got any hot water though. I'm sure that we were paying for their electricity downstairs. If we wanted a bath, (and let's face it, living in this squalor you would want one every half hour), then we had to boil up kettles of water and mix it with the cold, so that the paint didn't come off and we wouldn't turn pink.

The cooker didn't work at all, apart from one ring. So all our meals were out of tins and cooked on this one ring. There was one problem though. The tin opener didn't work. Julie and Kathy nominated me to go down to see Mr. Hanson about it. I knocked on his door and told him that the tin opener didn't work.

He glared at me and said, 'You must 'ave broke it. It was all right before you lot come 'ere. Your not 'avin' my tin opener to break. Gis yer tin. I'll open it.'

Therefore, whenever we wanted a tin opened, I had to go down and ask him to do it. I'm surprised he didn't charge us extra for this facility.

When I first saw the curtains in the living room, I thought that they were made of lace. They weren't of course. They were just full of holes. If they were moth holes, then the moths must have been the size of a bat. We might as well have not drawn them at night, as anyone standing out side could see in just as easily as if we had not. If someone looked in, he would probably think it was a crack house. Every cupboard looked like someone had been ill in them. There was dried sick everywhere. We had to take the blankets down the launderette to have them cleaned before we could use them, as they were covered in dried sick and diarrhoea.

We plugged the kettle in the next day and there was a firework display around the socket. Once again, the other two nominated me to go and see Mr. Hanson. He opened the door, I told him about the kettle, and he said, 'On no. You 'aven't broke sumink else, 'ave yer? It was all right before you come 'ere.' With that, he shut the door, and I was left standing with this portable death trap. We had to boil up pans of water on the stove after that.

One morning I was feeling quite ill, (just for a change), so Julie kindly boiled up a pan of water and made me a cup off coffee. She opened my bedroom door and it promptly came off in her hand. There was Julie, coffee in one hand, door in the other, with a look of disbelief on her face. I was volunteered once more to go down and face the dreaded Hanson man. 'Oh no, not you again. Wot 'ave yer broke nah?' he snarled.

I tried to explain to him that it came off in my sister's hand and that she wasn't practising her karate on it.

'Well it was all right before you lot come,' he said, 'you're wrecking my 'oliday flat.'

I know, we should have turned around and gone straight home. However, none of us had much money and we were all desperate for a holiday. Besides, I didn't want to face Dad and tell him that we forfeited all that money for nothing.

On the last day of our holiday, we had to get out of the flat by 10am. However, our train back wasn't until the afternoon, so I knocked on the Hanson's door to see if we could leave our cases in the flat for a couple of hours so that we didn't have to cart them around the town with us. I breathed a sigh of relief when Mrs. Hanson opened the door. She said that it would be OK to do that, and that we could hold on to the key until

we went. So we thanked her and went off for the day. When we came back in the afternoon for our cases, we decided to go to the toilet before we went. Just then, Mr. Hanson opened the door.
He said, 'What the hell are you lot doin' 'ere? I fort I saw the back of you lot. I've got ten minutes clean this place up before the next lot come.'

The only way anyone could clean that place up in ten minutes would be to use dynamite. We told him that his wife said we could leave our cases there, and now we had come to collect them.
'Well take yer bags and sling yer 'ook,' he snapped, 'I've 'ad enough of you lot.'
We slung our hooks, glad to see the back of the place. I loved Westgate and I will certainly go back there one day. But next time, I'll make sure the accommodation is fit for human habitation.

The following year Julie, Kathy and I decided to go to Cambridge. We hoped to get a similar accommodation to when we went to Oxford. However, we couldn't get in a student accommodation this time, so we had to stay in a guesthouse. This time, instead of the three of us sharing a place for twelve, we had to share a place designed for one. It was minuscule. They had squeezed in three beds in a single room. It was so small that the bedroom door wouldn't open fully. It was lucky that none of us was fat. We had to go outside to change our minds. If the person in the bed nearest the window wanted to go to the toilet during the night, they had to climb over the other two. I took the bed nearest the door. Partly because I always have to go during the night, but also I was used to being walked over.

The flat had en-suite, if you can call it that. It was a converted broom cupboard, comprising of a shower, toilet and sink. It was so cramped that you could almost go to the toilet while you were having a shower. It's no exaggeration, but the basin was so small that you could only wash one hand at a time in it. There was no room to hang a towel, so once you had your shower you had to shout out, and someone would put their hand round the door and hand you one. There was not even any room for soap. You had to take it in there with you.

The owner told us that there was tea and coffee making facilities. Well, she wasn't lying as such. There were indeed 3 tea bags and 3 teaspoons full of coffee. There were also three sachets of powdered milk, so you had to choose whether to have milk in your tea or your coffee. There was no sugar. Therefore, although we couldn't actually have her under the trade descriptions act, she came pretty close to the wire.

Whenever we went on holiday, we always went on the Guide Friday bus, to get our bearings. I recommend this to anyone on holiday in England, as it's a good way of finding out what you want to visit. Having decided what we wanted to see, we got off the bus and walked along the lanes in Cambridge, looking at all the colleges. We always had a large number of bags with us, as if we were going hiking through the jungle of Borneo. We took extra clothes in case it got cold, we took our packed lunches and as Kathy suffered various allergies in those days, she took the entire stock of Boots the Chemist, in case she was stung or got struck by lightening or something.

We had to cross the road, so I crossed first and Kathy followed me a few seconds later. Because I had looked for traffic, Kathy felt that she didn't have to bother. Just then, a student on a bike came round the corner at speed and ran into her. She was knocked to the floor and suffered a cut above her eyebrow. In those days Kathy was a bit of a hypochondriac, so as soon as she noticed blood seeping out of her head, that was it. She thought she was dying and had brain damage and was going off alarmingly. You would have thought that she had just been run over by a Chieftain tank.

The building on the corner of the road where the accident happened was being renovated. The builders working there heard the commotion and came running up to help. The foreman, a big, burly man, immediately started giving orders to his underlings. To one of them he said, 'You, go and get a chair for the lady.' The lackey duly ran in and brought out a folding chair, which he erected for Kathy to sit on. To another lackey the foreman said, 'Right, you go and get a cup of tea for the lady.' I didn't know at the time that you're not supposed to let people drink if they've had an accident, just in case they need surgery. The second lackey came out with what was the biggest mug of tea I have seen in my life. I didn't know if Kathy was supposed to drink it or do twenty lengths in it. It was so large and heavy that she couldn't hold it. So, Julie held it for her under her nose, as if it were a vapour inhaler.

The road this happened on was very narrow, as many are in Cambridge. It was narrower than usual, due to the scaffolding of the building work jutting out, which was why the cyclist didn't see Kathy in time. As quite a crowd had built up by now, you can imagine what the congestion was like. Cars were building up in both directions. There was my friend Kathy sitting precariously on a fold up chair in the middle of the road, dripping blood into a cauldron of tea, surrounded by numerous onlookers.

I was doing my best trying to stem the flow of blood with a paper hanky, when a car stopped next to us and a man got out, which just added to the obstruction. He was a travelling salesman, and he said that he had a first aid kit in his car. He got his first aid kit out and started treating Kathy. Meanwhile, Bob the Builder had called for an ambulance on his mobile phone. The ambulance arrived along with the police. They wanted to know why the whole of Cambridge had come to a standstill.

The paramedics started treating Kathy in readiness to take her to the ambulance. While this was happening, a policewoman asked me what had happened. I told her, and she had a word with the cyclist and allowed him to leave. The policewoman said it wasn't his fault or Kathy's fault. It was because the builders had their scaffolding too far out into the road and thus obstructing the vision. She then went to have a word with them.

The ambulance driver then said to me, 'Are you coming with us love, because we're going now?' I could see Kathy and Julie already sitting in the ambulance and I sure didn't want to be left alone. I didn't know where they were going and I thought that if they drove off without me, I would probably never see them again. So I climbed into the back off the ambulance with the ambulance man, Kathy, Julie and four hundredweight of bags. Just as the ambulance man shut the door, our last view of the scene was of this policewoman berating Bob the Builder and pointing to him and then pointing to us, and him shouting back at her, 'No, I'm not having that. I was only helping them. It wasn't my fault.'

We drove off and breathed a sigh of relief. We were glad that we weren't around to bear the brunt of Bob the Builder's anger at thinking that we had blamed him for the accident, when all he had done was help us.

The ambulance technician told us that they were taking us to Addenbrooke's hospital. During the journey, he asked Kathy various questions, but I had to answer for her as she kept passing out whenever she saw her blood. I don't know if he knew who was speaking, as it was hard to see anyone over the pile of bags in the ambulance.

We eventually got to accident and emergency at Addenbrooke's. They carried Kathy in, while Julie and I got all our bags out of the ambulance and struggled in with them, looking, for all intents and purposes, like we had just got off the boat. It must have looked as if we were moving in. We went over to the reception desk to explain what had happened. The receptionist said to me, 'There's going to be a long delay, I'm afraid, as we're decorating the waiting area. But in the meantime you can help us by choosing the colour scheme.'

It was bizarre, but absolutely true. I said to her, 'Well all right, but don't you want Kathy's details?'

'Oh yes', she said, 'but before I take her details, have a look at this colour chart. You see,' she carried on, 'you've just come through the door, so we would like your advice. Which colour do you think would be the most soothing?'

Well, I thought the most soothing thing would be to have Kathy seen, never mind what colour the walls were painted. Anyway, Kathy was deposited in the waiting area and we went over to join her, bringing all our bags with us, which meant that there was hardly any room for anyone else to get in. The nurse checked Kathy over and said that she wasn't too bad and that she only needed three stitches. She said that we would have to wait, as there were many urgent cases to see first. Mind you, as soon as Kathy heard that she had to have stitches, she nearly had a heart attack and got to the front of the queue.

Kathy obviously thought she was worse than she was, and even told me that she thought she was dying. I thought, oh, that's good. I take my friend on holiday and she comes back dead. She'll never let me hear the end of it.

While we were waiting there, the receptionist kept coming over to us and shoving various colour charts in front of my nose. I was getting fed up with this by now. I just wanted Kathy to be seen so that we could get out of there. I wasn't interested in choosing the colour for the waiting room. With any luck, I would never see it again. Nevertheless, she insisted. First, she wanted to know what basic colour it should be, and then what actual shade of that colour. If they did it the colour of my face, it would be puce.

Then she showed us a large book full of prints. She wanted to know which pictures they should hang, once the room was painted. Overall, we were there about 6 hours. She was lucky we didn't hang her on the wall.

We finally got home to our digs exhausted. I don't think anyone used the toilet during the night. None of us had the strength to climb over the others to get there. We did nothing the next day, as Kathy felt queasy and we were all tired, but the day after we all felt fit enough to go on a guided tour. Once more we loaded up our bags, (Kathy made sure she had all her paraphernalia for her delicate situation, from mosquito repellent to spare bandages to a defibrillator machine) and set off.

The guide took us to various parts of Cambridge, but one of the parts she took us was right opposite the building where Kathy had her accident two days earlier. The building was still going on, although to a smaller degree. Most of the scaffolding had been moved, so they could only work on one part at a time. We could see Bob the Builder standing there, shouting his orders to his underlings. We were terrified that he would see us, as I'm sure he would have come over and tackled us about grassing him up to the police and curtailing most of his work. Therefore, cowards as we were, we went and hid behind a wall until the tour moved on.

The rest of the holiday went without a hitch, and we all really enjoyed it. I know that Kathy dined out for years on how she cheated death and had to have major surgery at a top teaching hospital.

KARL

One afternoon to get out of the flat, I went for a walk to Fleetville, which was about a mile away. I wandered into various shops just to look around. I found that when my mind was in turmoil, window-shopping often calmed me down. I ended up in a newsagent's, just to look at the magazines on the shelves. Although I could never settle at home to read, (which was one of my biggest regrets, as I loved reading), I liked looking at the magazines in these shops.

Perusing the shelves, I came across a magazine that made me do a double take. I thought the person on the front of the magazine looked familiar. I looked in disbelief at what I saw. It was Karl! I had not seen him since that day in Ruskin Park when he was attending the outpatient's clinic at the Maudsley. The photo of him was terrible. He looked very emaciated and gaunt and he had obviously lost a lot of weight. His photo was on one side of the cover and on the other side was a photo of another man of normal weight. It was like the before and after photos in weight watching magazines, except in reverse. I can't remember the exact wording now, but the caption under Karl said something like, 'This man is dying of Anorexia. He has no hope.' Under the photo of the other man the caption read, 'This man could have ended up like Karl if he hadn't pulled himself together and overcome Anorexia.'

I thought that was an awful portrayal. The magazine had written Karl off and more or less blamed him for his illness. You can't compare one person's illness with another's. Everyone is different. I bought the magazine and took it home to read. The main thrust of it was about how everyone knew that girls suffered from Anorexia but maybe they didn't know that it also affected men to some degree. Inside the article concentrated on three men. Two of them had suffered from Anorexia but were now 'cured' and living a normal life. The other story was about the man for which there was no hope. That was Karl. Even though Karl was obviously very thin, the way the photograph was taken made him look even worse. It was a much-sensationalised article and I thought that it was a bad piece of journalism. I later found out that the person who put the magazine in touch with Karl was the man that I had met on my first day in the Maudsley, the TV producer.

I was shocked at the article, and the part of me that roots for the underdog came to the fore. I immediately wanted to help him. I really liked Karl when we were in hospital together, and he always talked to me like a friend. Deep down I suppose that I wanted to rekindle the friendship that we had. I didn't think that I would have much chance, after all, who would want to be friends with me? Anyway, I took courage in both hands, and went to the phone box to phone him at his parents' house where he lived. I was terrified of talking to him, as I was terrified of speaking to any man. The fear of rejection was overwhelming. He picked up the phone and I explained who I was, and like before, he spoke to me as if I was the one person in the world that he wanted to talk to.

We spoke for a while and caught up on old times. He said that he went on holiday the year before with Yasmin and Clare, (the girls who lived in the annex on my ward), and was seeing someone else now who he had met at the Maudsley. Her name was Leanne, and she lived in Faversham in Kent. Leanne at one time was an anorexic, but she now binge ate. She was normal weight by this time, but she felt that she looked obese. Therefore, she wouldn't leave her house unless her parents drove her. Both families became quite friendly, meeting up at Christmas and birthdays. Leanne was to become important to my story later on.

Karl came across on the phone that everything was fine in his life, although as before, we never really talked about his illness. However, he did tell me that they had tricked him about the magazine article. It was supposed to be an article about educating people on the facts of Anorexia, and they said that they wanted his side of the story as to why he couldn't eat.

We agreed that I would phone him again the following week, and I floated back to my flat after the success of the phone call. I lived on the euphoria for the next few days and worked towards the next time I would call him, such was my sad life. This carried on for three or four weeks, but then one day when I rang, his mum Kay answered the phone. Wherein Karl had always put on a brave front when he spoke to me, I got a different perspective from Kay. She asked me if Karl had told me that he now weighed only seven and a half stone. Of course, he hadn't and I was shocked to hear this news. For someone who stood six foot two, seven and a half stone was skeletal. She said that sometimes he would go with her to the shops but that he had to come home after a short time, as he didn't have the strength to walk.

Kay told me that Karl was an outpatient at the Gordon Hospital in Victoria. The regime at the Maudsley did nothing for Karl, (or for the majority of other Anorexics), so his GP and the community nurse put him in touch with the Gordon. A wonderful psychiatric nurse-cum-counsellor called David Britten headed the Anorexic department of the Gordon Hospital. David Britten's attitude to dealing with Anorexia was poles apart from the factory farm, which was the Maudsley. He realised that you had to work with the patients and with the illness inside, which would hopefully lead the patients to eat of their own free will.

Kay told me that Karl was going back to the Gordon the next day with his dad, Tom. She said that she was worried what was going to happen, as they had told Karl on his last visit that if he hadn't put on any weight by the next appointment, they would have to section him under the mental health act. Of course, I knew none of this. When Kay put Karl on, I questioned him about it. 'Oh it's nothing,' he said, 'it's only going to be a check up. I'll be back home in the afternoon.' He wasn't!

I phoned his house the next day to see how he had got on. Kay answered the phone and was very distressed. She said that when they had seen Karl and saw how thin he was, they knew that they couldn't let it go any more. Karl was becoming a danger to himself. David Britten, Karl's dad and a doctor, sat in a room for three hours trying to persuade Karl to admit himself voluntarily. Unfortunately, Karl wasn't having any of it and so they had no choice but to section him.

I asked Kay if it would be all right for me to ring her every few days for a progress report and she agreed. During these phone calls, Kay told me that Karl refused to eat anything in hospital and would only drink black coffee. His weight was falling by the day. He became so thin that he had pressure sores all over his body, where he had no fat to pad him. He had to sit on a fur rug to try to ease the problem, and he would carry this rug wherever he went. He didn't go far I hasten to add, as his legs would hardly carry him. They really expected Karl to die and they had a crash team standing by in case he went into cardiac arrest, which he could have done at any time. David Britten had gone through with Karl about the signs he would get if he was about to die, and that he should press the emergency button if he got any of the signs.

Kay told me that Karl would like to see me. I didn't want to push myself, as I felt that no one would like to see me. Therefore, I told her that I would wait until I heard from Karl personally, before I went there. In any case, I didn't think that I could handle it, as things seemed so bad. I had watched people I was close to in the Maudsley die and I didn't want to see another one.

About four days later, I received a postcard from Karl asking me to go in and see him. How he even had the strength to write the card is a miracle. In contrast to how things really were, he wrote the card like a 'wish you were here' holiday postcard. Once again, he was in denial of his illness. He wrote that it would be very nice to see me, as he was quite bored and that he didn't have much to do. The fact that he was at death's door wasn't mentioned.

I was very nervous about going to see Karl, but at the same time excited. Apart from anything else, it was an outing for me. Anything that got me out of my flat was worthwhile. When I walked onto the ward and saw him, I was shocked. He looked like the pictures you see of victims from the concentration camps. He was in a bad way, even compared to many of the patients I had seen in the Maudsley. He was the same person inside though, and once more made me feel like I was the one person in the world that he wanted to see. We went into a side room, and his mum and dad were there, which was the first time I had met them. They were very nice, ordinary people.

Karl's mum was agoraphobic and so was unable to visit on her own and found it hard even with her husband Tom. She was also addicted to the drug Ativan, which she took for her high anxiety. This drug made her feel sedated all the time. Tom was a commissionaire at the BBC. He hadn't been well lately but everyone assumed that was because he was worrying about Karl and being by his bedside every day. What no one realised at the time was that Tom had terminal cancer.

We had a nice afternoon together, and we all got on well. Tom went and got us all a cup of coffee, and when he came back, he told us that there was a girl in the kitchen eating something out of a dog bowl on the floor. He was quite shocked about this and said to me, 'There's some terribly ill people here Sue.' I had to agree, and his son was one of them.

Although I was afraid of most men at the time, I wasn't afraid of Karl. Primarily, that was because he was nice to me, but also because he was no threat. He was dressed in a dressing gown sitting on a fur rug, hanging on to life. Therefore, I asked him if he would like me to visit him the following week, and he said yes please, so we agreed that I would. Visiting Karl for the weeks and months to come was to become the high spot of the week for me.

As the weeks went on, Karl's condition got worse. After about the second or third time that I went to see him, he was in a different bed with curtains round him. The hospital had decided to start a punishment regime in an effort to get him to eat of his own accord. They stopped him from seeing his parents, because they felt that his dependency on them had to be broken. Anorexia is often coupled with the relationship of the patient's family and their over possessiveness. The hospital wanted to be the controlling influence, rather than Karl's parents. Therefore, I was the only visitor Karl got. I think that the only reason they let me in was because I had a coat similar to what the nurses wore. I think I may have been mistaken for a nurse, just as I was on my first night in the Maudsley.

One day I was sitting there talking to Karl, when a nurse came up to him and told him that he had a phone call. He went off to answer it and came back an hour later. 'That was a surprise', he said, 'that was Leanne.'

I'll say it was a surprise. He told me that he wasn't allowed any phone calls. That was the first of the lies that Karl would tell me. Of course, I wasn't to know this at the time. I had a lot to learn and I learned the hard way I learned the hard way.

Karl's stay in hospital lasted about a year and I visited him once a week. In the meantime, I realised that I had to do something constructive with my life. I wanted to try to get back to some kind of work. I went to the local job centre and saw a woman who was an expert in getting people who were on benefit back to the workplace. I realised that I was no good in an office environment, or anything that involved a lot of stress or pressure. I would still have liked to be a teacher, although I realised that it was not possible. However, it was possible that I could be a classroom assistant.

After attending various workshops and seminars, I eventually heard about an NVQ course at Oakland's College. This course was specifically for older women who had been out of the work environment for a while or who wanted a change of career. It was a 'back to study' course, but without the pressure of a formal college education. At the end of the course, you got an NVQ 1, 2 and 3 in general caring, which would then allow you to work in an old people's home or work with the mentally handicapped.

I enrolled on this course, which involved doing one day a week at Oakland's for lectures, one day a week for home study and writing essays based on the lectures, and the other three days were for work experience. Fortunately, they had two departments at Oakland's. One was for working with mentally handicapped adults and the other department was for slow learners and adult literacy. I felt that I would like work in the adult literacy class. However, when I went along for the interview, I found out that the course I was on wouldn't give me the qualifications needed for this work. I was referred to the special needs department. I had an interview there, and they said that they would take me on for the three days a week during my course.

This was a very happy time for me. Although I found the course work quite hard, (as my brain was still sluggish with the illness and the drugs), I thoroughly enjoyed the work at Oakland's, especially the Friday cookery classes with Chris, Jill, and Dot. These three women were very nice to me and were to figure more in my life later on. I loved the students as they took me for what I was, not what I should have been. At last, I had found something that I felt I could do. Although I still had all my health problems, the time I spent doing the work experience was a real boost to my confidence and I absolutely loved it.

During this time, I carried on seeing Karl on a weekly basis. I was pleased to see that during that year, he was looking better and better and had put on weight. One particular day I arrived on the ward and was surprised to see him up, dressed, shaved and looking well. He suggested that we went out for a coffee, as he was allowed off the ward now. I had to face some of my fears now. You see, while

I was visiting him and he was a vulnerable person in a hospital bed, it was safe. Now he was dressed and looking normal, he was a man again. I still had that irrational fear of men. I suppose I felt more vulnerable myself, and had a fear of rejection. Now that he wasn't a captive audience, he could choose not to see me any more. I felt that while I was the only one that visited him, he had no choice but to see me. After all, I was better than nothing. Now that he had a choice, I feared that I would no longer have a role. I still felt attracted to Karl, and obviously more so now that he was fit and well. However, he was more attractive to the other girls as well. Why would he want to have anything to do with boring, ugly Susan Kennedy, when he could have his pick? Nevertheless, I agreed to go out for coffee, and we found a place round the corner.

While we sat sipping our coffees, he told me that he was soon to be moving to a homeless hostel in Victoria. He said it was the hospital's idea. The idea was that any anorexic that lived at home with his or her parents, were thought to have a better chance of recovery away from that possible parental influence. Karl's parents were against this idea as they wanted him home with them, but Karl thought it was a good idea to become more independent. He would still be attending the Gordon as an inpatient for counselling and meals, but it would be easy for him to get there, as he would be living round the corner.

The building Karl moved into was enormous, reminiscent of an old Victorian workhouse. It housed over two hundred people in tiny, single rooms. There was just enough room for a bed, a wardrobe and a small chest of drawers. All sorts of undesirables lived in this hostel. Drug addicts and alcoholics were by far the largest contingent, with a few rooms given over for patients from the Gordon. There was a filthy kitchenette at the end of each corridor, with a kettle if anyone wanted a hot drink. The kettle was chained to the wall. Not only that, but in the communal toilets the toilet paper was also chained to the wall. That just about sums up the place.

Once Karl moved into the hostel, I came down once a week and we spent the day in London. Neither of us had much money, so we could only go to the free places, for example art galleries, but we still enjoyed ourselves. It was certainly the high spot of my week.

Around this time, I had finished my years NVQ courses and my work experience. I was offered the chance to work on a summer scheme, which was run for the mentally handicapped adults. This involved various trips out on minibuses for picnics in the country or occasionally trips to the seaside. These trips were a lot of fun, and I thoroughly enjoyed participating in them. One such day trip was to Southend. We travelled in convoy of three minibuses and a couple of cars. Our minibus was at the back. On the way to the seaside, it broke down and I watched all the others disappear into the sunset, leaving us there.

We called the AA out and they got it going again, and we finally arrived in Southend about two hours after the others. On the way home, one of the tutors followed us in her car, just in case we broke down again. We did. This time the AA man said that there was no hope. The minibus had finally gone to the big garage in the sky.

The minibus was loaded onto the back of the pickup truck and we put as many students as we could into the tutor's car. The rest of them came with me in the front of the pickup truck, which could carry six passengers. The AA mechanic was a big bruiser of a man who was quite capable of dealing with broken down vehicles. He wasn't so used to dealing with broken down people. He was warily looking through his rear view mirror, watching all these emotionally traumatised students behaving in bizarre way. Some of them cried all the way home, yet others wanted to kiss and cuddle the mechanic. He kept saying, 'Keep them away from me. Don't let them kiss me.' I was obviously used to students showing their feelings outwardly. That's just their way; they won't think twice about cuddling someone who they like. This poor man wasn't used to it, and I had to try to keep the students away from him in order for us to get home safely.

We eventually got back to the central home, where many of the students lived. However, others lived in their own home, so Chris and I started ferrying them to their respective houses. All the addresses where these students lived were locked away in the college. Luckily, most of them knew where they lived and so it was quite easy to take them home. All but one chap, that is.

We knew he lived in Harpenden, but that was the limit of our knowledge. Consequently, we drove round and round Harpenden in the hopes that he recognised somewhere. We got to the main shopping area and asked him if he knew where he was. He said, 'Um, I think my mummy brought me down here once.' So off we went again. This went on for hours, until quite by chance he pointed to a man and said, 'I know that man.'

The rubber from the wheels sent up a black cloud as we screeched to a halt in front of this passer by. We got out of the minibus and walked over to the man who probably thought that we were a hit squad. When we asked him if he knew the little chap in our bus, he breathed a sigh of relief and said, 'Oh yes, I know him. That's Douglas; he lives next door to me'. Sighs of relief all round as we finally delivered our last charge back home safely.

One day during the summer scheme, I was asked to take a student up to London to get a copy of his birth certificate for him. I did this, but on the way back I decided to do a bit of a detour and call in at the Gordon Hospital to say hello to Karl. I should not have done this, but in those days I was obsessed with Karl, and I wanted to see more of him. I waited at the entrance at the set time, but there was no sign of him. Just then, two girls who lived at the hostel with Karl, Nicky and Mary, came out of the dining area. I asked them if they had seen Karl and they looked at each other rather sheepishly. They told me that Karl didn't go there for his meals. This came as a shock to me, as he told me that he had all his meals there. I had caught him out in yet another lie, a trait that would continue for all the time that I knew him.

Karl and three of the girls who lived in the hostel with him, Nicky, Mary and Sylvia, had arranged to go and see Joseph and the Amazing Technicolor Dreamcoat at the London Palladium. At the last minute, Sylvia pulled out, so Karl asked me if I would like to go. His parents had paid for my ticket as a thank you for all the help and support I had given him.

Because it was on late at night, there was a problem for me getting home afterwards. However, Karl's parents said that I could stay over at their house in Acton, West London. I was so excited. I was going to actually go out with Karl and then stay at his house overnight. I met Karl at the tube station and we went on from there to meet the others in the theatre.

We enjoyed the show and then afterwards the two girls went off together and Karl took me back to his parents place. Walking along together, I desperately wanted to hold his hand. I wanted to bring the relationship on a stage further. Up until then we had just been friends, but I wanted more. On the other hand, in my fragile state, I couldn't risk rejection. So we just carried on as friends, with this feeling burning away inside me.

Tom and Kay made me feel very welcome at their home. It was a very humble house, (the landlord they had did no repairs or renovation, so the place was in some disarray) but they did their best and it was very homely. Tom went off to work, (he was on nights) and Kay and I went off to bed. Karl stayed downstairs. I later found out that he had a heavy eating binge that night, although I was oblivious to that part of his problem at that time.

The next morning there was no sign of him, so I had breakfast with Kay. Tom came home from his night shift so I said goodbye to him before he went to bed. About midday, Karl finally emerged. There was no mention of what happened the night before.

Karl's parents knew about his eating binges, but they didn't talk to me about them at the time. In that respect, they were very much like my mum and dad, and kept everything quiet.

Karl took me to the station and I made my way home to Martins Court. I remember thinking on my way home, how 'safe' his house was. It reminded me of my family home, with his mum and dad similar in nature to my parents. I felt that I didn't want to leave. I liked the safety and security, which I never had in my flat.

My time was now taken up with working at the school weekdays, (I was now a full time assistant), combined with Friday Folk on Friday evenings and the Mass Centre Sunday Mornings. The rest of Sunday, I spent with Karl. From time to time my friend Kathy would come and stay for a weekend, Julie would join us, and we'd do something together.

Come October, Karl told me that Sylvia had asked him to go on holiday with her to Ireland, to stay with her relatives. He said that he didn't want to go but she had begged him as she was nervous about going on her own. He said that he didn't want to let her down, so agreed. I hadn't met Sylvia at this time, but later on when I did, I realised that she was hardly the nervous type. Many things I only heard from Karl's point of view, but as time went on, I learnt to read between the lines.

From what I could gather from the trip, Sylvia's relatives knew that she was anorexic but, according to Karl, she told them that he was her boyfriend and that he didn't have an eating disorder. As time went on, I realised that I couldn't believe half of what Karl told me, so I don't know if he thought of himself as Sylvia's boyfriend or was just masquerading to please her.

Because Sylvia's relatives didn't know about Karl's anorexia, they served him full size meals, which they expected him to eat. When he came home, he had put on about two stone. This completely freaked him out and made his problem even worse. He lost the weight as soon as he could. I later found out from Sylvia that Karl also had a drink problem. Although the way he put it, it was Sylvia who made him drink. He always had an excuse.

After the holiday, things between Karl and I stayed pretty much the same. At the beginning of December, I invited him to my flat. I was so nervous about it that I invited Julie and Kathy as well. That was the first time Julie and Kathy had met Karl.

Karl and I had been seeing each other for around two years by this time, and we were good friends, but I wanted things to move on a stage. I bought him a Christmas card and I wrote inside how I felt about him and that I would like us to be more than just friends. We went up to London just before Christmas to an art gallery and I gave him the card then, but I asked him not to open it until 25th December. However, as the day progressed I started to have second thoughts. I thought that if he didn't feel the same way that I did, it would ruin our friendship. I felt that I would rather see him as a friend than not at all. I decided that I would ask for the card back, as I was sure that if he read it, everything we had going would end.

While we were sitting on St Pancras station waiting for my train, I spun him a lie. I told him that I had put his card in the wrong envelope, and that he had my dad's card. Karl turned round to me and said, 'It's too late. I've opened the card already.' That's all he said. He didn't comment on it at all. I didn't say anything either. What could I say? I didn't want to make things worse than they already were. We stood together in an awkward silence until my train came, then I got on and we waved each other goodbye. I was convinced that that would be the last time I would see him.

I heard nothing from him at all over the Christmas period. I had a terrible time, berating myself for being such an idiot. I wanted a life; I wanted to go out and about. I had ruined everything. Whatever made me think that someone as good looking as Karl would want any kind of a relationship with me? In fact, why would anyone want any kind of a relationship with me? I was worthless, ugly and a waste of space. Such was the low opinion I had of myself.

On New Years Day, I got a phone call from Karl. He told me to expect a card through the post in which he had replied to my card. We were due to meet on 4th January to visit the Imperial War Museum. I didn't mention this to him, as I was sure that he would tell me it was over in his card. Every day when the postman came, I ran to the door to see if the card had arrived. It finally arrived on the fourth, the day of the trip. I opened the card in trepidation, as if it was my A level results. I couldn't believe what I read. He said that he felt the same way about me as I felt about him, but he had been too nervous to tell me. He said that he wanted us to become an item. I was elated and excited, but at the same time scared. This was what I had always wanted.

I went up to London and met Karl at Kings Cross Thameslink. He looked very smart. I was so nervous that I was shaking. He took my hand and all my nerves disappeared. We walked hand in hand round the museum, but I could hardly take in my surroundings. I felt as though I was floating on air. I not only had a boyfriend, but I had a good-looking one with a great personality that all the other girls fancied. I was I heaven.

He told me that he wrote the card to me soon after he had received mine, but lost his nerve about posting it. He said that he was invited to a New Years Eve party, and although he wasn't one for parties, his friend persuaded him to go. He said that just to get through the ordeal of the party he got drunk, (at that time, I didn't know that he had a drink problem anyway). Anyhow, having got some Dutch courage inside him, he plucked up the nerve to post the card. I was glad that he did. I floated home that night, after a wonderful day; the day that I fell in love for the first time.

For our next outing, we had planned to meet up with Nicky, one of the girls from the hostel. Nicky was a wonderful artist, and she wanted to go and see a Toulouse Lautrec exhibition. After the exhibition, Nicky went home and Karl and I went and sat on a bench by the Southbank. Karl looked at me, took my face in his hands, and gently kissed me. It was freezing cold that day and I was shivering, although not from the cold. Things were looking up for me. I was infatuated with Karl and he told me he felt the same. I had no reason to doubt him, and I didn't want to doubt him. However, on our next meeting, a few doubts did creep in.

On that occasion, we went for a walk round St James' park then afterwards we went back to his room in the hostel. I got the feeling that he didn't really want me there. He kept saying that he didn't want me to get tired after our long walk and then he said that he would be worried about me going home in the dark. He never worried in the past about my going home when it was dark. I couldn't fathom it out. While we sat in his room, he kept looking at his watch and saying that it might be safer for me if I went home by seven.

Just before 7o'clock there was a knock at the door. Karl looked sheepishly at me and went to answer it. I couldn't see who it was as he only opened the door a crack and stood between the door and me. I could hear though. It was Sylvia, and it was obvious from what I could hear, that they had arranged to meet. I picked up from the way they were talking that it was different from his friendship with Nicky. This was more clandestine, like boyfriend and girlfriend. I heard him say, 'Well, you know, it's a bit difficult. I have someone here at the moment. Can we make it later?'

'Oh yes,' she said, 'who have you got with you?' and with that, she shoved the door open and pushed Karl out of the way. I smiled innocently at her, and said hello. She shot daggers at me, and if looks could kill, I wouldn't be writing this now. From the look she gave me, it was obvious that she regarded me as a rival. She turned to Karl and said, 'No, I won't be coming back later.' She then turned on her heels and stormed out. Karl went running down the corridor after her saying, 'Wait a minute, wait a minute, let me explain.'

In my innocence, I didn't know what to make of it. After a while, Karl came back and told me that he had arranged to see Sylvia that evening to try to help her with her eating problem. Well, that didn't quite ring true with me. If it was so innocent, why didn't he tell me about it? Why did Sylvia look at me like something she had scraped off her foot?

Going back home on the tube later, I challenged Karl about it. I accused him of seeing Sylvia behind my back and that he was playing one off against the other. He swore blind that he wasn't. He said that Sylvia had a crush on him and that she wanted things to develop between them, but he said that he didn't feel the same way about her. He said that she kept pestering him and he only spoke to her to keep the peace. I left it at that. I suppose that I wanted to believe him.

The next day he phoned me and he said that when he went for his meals at the Gordon, (another lie? I don't know), Sylvia shunned him. He also said that all the other girls were refusing to talk to him, and he couldn't understand what he had done wrong. He said that it proved how sick Sylvia was, because she had built this fantasy in her head and turned everyone against him. He protested his innocence and because I loved him, I believed him. They say that love is blind and I was certainly very short sighted. However, as I got to know Karl over time, my 'eyesight' improved.

I was to have an emotional roller-coaster ride with Karl over the next few years. I loved him and I tried to help him, but I was unwell myself. His lies and deceits combined with his self-destructive illness, took its toll on me. I had no idea what I was letting myself in for.

MORE COLOURFUL CHARACTERS AT OAKLANDS.

My job at Oakland's was my small contribution into rehabilitating the mentally handicapped for a life on their own. The hospitals were starting to close and the patients were moving out into smaller homes. When I started at Oakland's, the transition period was already well underway. The hospitals were huge places, like mini towns. It was no small feat moving everyone away. Many of the inpatients would go to workshops in the hospital grounds and do simple packing jobs, (much as I had to do in the Maudsley), others worked as gardeners on the grounds and some worked in the kitchens.

As the hospitals were closing, so these workshops were also running down. In order to give the patients something to do and to prepare them for the outside world, departments within colleges like mine were set up for the task. I loved my job at the college. It was as near to teaching as I could get, but apart from that, I knew that I was doing a valuable job in helping the students come to terms with life on their own. We ran literacy and numeracy classes, gardening classes, art classes, drama classes, and reminiscent classes for the elderly. My favourite subject though, was cookery.

Some of the students were quite familiar to me from my time at Cell Barnes Mass centre. Andrew Unsworth to name but one. I have mentioned Andrew before. He was the industrious one at the Mass centre who would wait until the end of the service and take money out of the collection plate. The first time I met Andrew, was during my fifth year at Nicholas Breakspear School. In the summer holiday, I volunteered to work at Cell Barnes on a summer scheme, helping to look after the younger patients.

One day in a painting class I handed Andrew some paints and brushes and told him to wait a minute while I went and got him some paper. I got the paper and came back; just in time to see the last bit of the paintbrush disappear into his mouth. He had eaten all the paints and all the brushes. He had even eaten the two yoghurt pots that he was supposed to wash the brushes in. Andrew ate anything and everything. I couldn't turn my back on him for a minute. No prizes for imagining my reaction when I found out that Andrew was to be a member of our cookery class at Oakland's.

Now, the students that came to the cookery classes were supposed to bring money for the ingredients, which the homes and hospitals provided. However, every time we asked Andrew for his money, he would say, 'No money lady. Got no money, 'ave I?'

We wondered about this, as all the other students had their money. The tutors even went so far as to phone his ward at Cell Barnes, to ask the ward nurse why Andrew never had any money. She said that he should have some money as they always gave it to him. Nevertheless, every Friday at cookery, I would go to Andrew to collect his money and I got the same answer, 'No money lady. Got no money, 'ave I?'

We couldn't understand why Andrew never had his money for cookery, until one day I was sitting eating my sandwiches, when I saw Andrew get off the minibus and head purposefully towards the refectory. I followed him down there and watched as he bought handfuls of chocolate then shovel it all into his mouth. I then went back to the cookery room and waited for him. I asked him if he had his cookery money, and once more got the reply, 'No money, lady. Got no money, 'ave I?' I let him know that his scheme had been rumbled, and after that, we got his cookery money direct from his hospital.

Mind you, that didn't stop him in his quest to eat anything and everything. This was a cookery class after all. Very little of Andrew's food got anywhere near an oven. He would shove most of it in his mouth raw. What's more, we couldn't leave the store cupboard unguarded if Andrew was doing cookery. He would go in and stuff his face with currents, raisins, flour, in fact everything. He would come out of the cupboard with his cheeks bulging like a hamsters, with flour and cooking chocolate smeared all over his face. He tried to look innocent, and swore blind that he hadn't been near the cupboard, but it didn't really work.

You couldn't help but like Andrew. He was very hyperactive and ran around a lot, but he had a big heart. If any of the other students got upset for any reason, Andrew would go up to them in his big, blustery way, and put his arm around them and say, 'Not worry. Be all right.'

He was also prone to having epileptic fits. One day he had a fit in the classroom. I wasn't trained in dealing with that kind of thing, but luckily, Chris and Jill were there and knew what to do. After someone has an epileptic fit it takes a while for them to come round properly. Andrew sat silently on the floor after his seizure, which was the first time I had seen him quiet. For the rest of the afternoon and in fact for the rest of the term, he came up to each of us in turn and said, 'Sorry, not my fault. Sorry.' We tried to reassure him that it wasn't his fault. Nevertheless, he kept repeating this for weeks, 'Sorry, had a fit. Not my fault. Still come to cookery?' It broke my heart.

Another character from the cookery class was a man called Brian. He lived in sheltered accommodation quite close to the college. Brian had lived a normal life until one day he was involved in a bad road accident, which had left him brain damaged. He was very enthusiastic about going to classes and was always smiling, but he could hardly speak, and so mostly used sign language. He could only say certain words and phrases, like, 'Not my fault, your fault' and, 'It's her fault', and 'Not worth it.' Another of Brian's catchphrases was, 'He died.' and he would then do the sign of the cross and imitate shovelling of the grave. He would use these phrases for everything. For example, if he saw you in the street, he would call out at the top of his voice, 'It's her fault.' and point straight at you. The looks I got from passers by when that happened would make a statue blush. If someone didn't turn up at college because they had a cold or something, Brian would reliably inform you, 'He died.' and do the sign of the cross and shovelling of the grave. One day, Peter, Brian's flatmate, didn't turn up for cookery.

'Where's Peter today, Brian?' I asked.

'He died.' said Brian, followed by the sign of the cross and the shovelling of the grave. You couldn't rely on Brian because according to him, quite a lot of people died each week.

Brian was quite limited at what he could and couldn't do, but he was able to do his own shopping, provided he was not put under any pressure. One day I was shopping in Tesco's, and found myself at the back of a long queue for the checkout. Everyone in the queue was tutting, sighing, and moaning about someone holding everyone up. When I looked at the front of the queue, I saw Brian standing there looking very flustered. As he only had a limited vocabulary, he found it hard to make himself understood.

The woman on the cash desk was trying to explain to Brian that there was an offer on one of the items he had bought, and that he could have another one free. Brian was having trouble understanding all this and was getting more and more worked up. Suddenly he looked to the back of the queue and spotted me standing there. His face brightened up and he pointed at me and shouted at the top of his voice, 'It's her fault.' Of course, everyone in the queue turned to look at me, wondering what I had done to this poor man at the front.

I rapidly went to the cash desk and sorted his problem out. As a bonus, the woman put my things through next so that I didn't have to go to the back of the queue. When he was happy, Brian would come out with his other catchphrase, 'Not worth it.' He was a lovely man.

I worked with dozens of different students during my time at Oakland's. They all had their own characteristics and quirks. They all gave me a lot of unconditional love. Occasionally, one or two students would come round to my flat after college, if they had particular difficulties coping on their own. I would show them how to pay bills or how to buy things from shops. It was quite upsetting to see some of them in flats on their own but unable to cope. I thought that it was unkind to do this to them. One man called Colin, had every cooking facility in his flat, but was unable to use any of it. Although he managed in the cookery class, when he was on his own he lost his confidence. He went to a local garage every day and bought cake and ice cream, and whenever he wasn't at college would have cake and ice cream for breakfast, dinner and tea.

Another man whose flat I visited didn't understand how the hot water system worked. Someone had told him to make sure that he turned the immersion heater off after he had a bath, because it cost a lot of money. He didn't want to get into trouble and so he never switched the immersion on. As a result, he had to wash in cold water.

The Care in the Community program was being implemented too quickly and without proper patient selection. You can't just put anyone into a flat and expect him or her to get on with it. Some of these people were quite old and had been in care all their lives. No one would ever suggest putting five and six year old children in a flat on their own and telling them to get on with it. There would be an outrage. Nevertheless, some of these people had a mental age of five or six. What's the difference? In my opinion, it was cruel.

A MOVING TIME FOR KARL

During this time, Karl was moved from the homeless hostel to a mother and baby unit in Maida Vale. This was the next step to getting him a place of his own. The idea of moving him to the mother and baby unit was that, because he shouldn't have been there and thus taking up a room needed for a single mother, he would be re-housed sooner. The mother and baby unit was a step up from the homeless hostel. There was slightly more space, and each room had a sink and cooking facilities. It was a bit like a studio flat.

Karl was also spending some time at my flat now. He only ever stayed a night or two, sleeping on the sofa bed downstairs, but I enjoyed his company. I felt more in control while he was there, my eating was more normal and I didn't feel so depressed.

One day I was alone in my flat and felt very down. I felt unable to cope and I was eating everything in sight. I knew that I had to get out. I didn't have work that day, so I decided to get on a train and go and see Karl in Maida Vale. I arrived at his place and knocked on the door, but when he opened it, he looked very shocked at seeing me there. I explained that I was having a bad day and that I couldn't cope on my own and needed his company. He was nice on the surface, but I could tell that he didn't want me there.

He said, 'Oh well, I have to go back to the Gordon Hospital for my meals.' This didn't ring true to me, as I knew that he didn't have to have his meals in the Gordon any more, and even when he was supposed to, he hardly turned up for them.

When I challenged him about this he said, 'Oh yes, well, I promised Sylvia that I would go back and support her eating her meal.' None of this sounded right to me, however I didn't say anything, but instead said that I would wait for him in his room as I couldn't go back to my flat.

I was exhausted due to the mental fatigue so he left me to sleep on his bed while he went off, supposedly, to support Sylvia at the Gordon. He came back late at night and he said that the reason he was so long was that it took Sylvia a long time to get through her meal. I didn't challenge him about it because that would have led to a row and then we would be finished. I needed the support of Karl, as I had no one else on the same wavelength as me who knew what I was going through. Of course, with hindsight, it was obvious that Karl was leading a double life. He was seeing Sylvia part of the week, and me the rest of the time, and never the twain shall meet. I knew there was nothing I could do about it. I wanted Karl in my life and would have done anything to keep him.

One day on an outing to Kenwood House in Hampstead, I found out that Karl wasn't just leading a double life; he was leading a triple life. Sitting on a bench at Kenwood, he turned to me and said, 'Mum says that I have to do something about Leanne. She keeps phoning me.'

It took me a minute to remember who Leanne was. She was the girl who 'unexpectedly' phoned him at the Gordon Hospital, while I was there.

'What do you mean?' I asked.

He said, 'Well, Leanne's got it into her head that we're an item. Her parents must be a bit twisted as well, because they all think that Leanne and I are engaged and that we're going to get married'.

I said, 'Well, how weird. Why would they think such a thing?'

He said, 'Well you see, while I wasn't well and was living at home, Leanne and I would phone each other, just to talk about our illnesses and for support. Occasionally her mum and dad brought her down and both families got friendly with each other.'

He went on, 'I also used to go down to see her in Faversham, and when I got there, her mother and father would leave us alone together, telling us that we needed time by ourselves. It was obvious that they saw us as a couple, and that we would naturally end up together. I didn't want to rock the boat by saying that we were only friends.'

Karl never wanted to rock the boat. I would later find out that he would say whatever anyone wanted to hear, just to keep the peace.

He said, 'I told Leanne that I was moving to a flat of my own, so she went out and bought me a pine bathroom set. Mum told me that I shouldn't really accept it if Leanne and I were not going to end up together.'

Well, this was how it was being presented to me. That it was all to do with Leanne's sickness and that it was all in her mind and that he didn't want to hurt her feelings, as she didn't have anyone else. I told Karl that it was ridiculous that someone should think that you were going to marry them just because you phoned each other for support. Of course, I didn't want to believe that there was something more to it than that. I only found out the truth later on in our relationship.

To cut a long story short, I found out much later from Kay, Karl's mum, that he was seeing almost as much of Leanne as he was me and that she phoned the family home most nights. So whenever I was out with Karl somewhere and Leanne rang, Karl's parents would have to make some excuse that he was staying at the hostel or something,

One day, I found a birthday card that Karl had written out to Leanne. It was not the kind of card that you would send a mere friend. It was a card you would send a lover.

When I challenged him about it, he said, 'Well, I didn't want to upset or hurt her. She doesn't have anyone else. I feel sorry for her because she's bought me all these presents for my flat and she thinks that we're going to end up together.'

I told Karl that he had to ring her and tell her the truth, and that it wasn't fair to keep stringing her along like this. He said that he would, but I later found out that he never did. Karl would never accept any responsibility for his life.

Karl's mum challenged me about it one day, thinking that I was a co-conspirator with this deception. She said that it wasn't fair on Leanne if she thought that Karl was going to be with her. I said to her that I thought that Karl had phoned Leanne and had sorted it all out. Kay said that he obviously hadn't, and that she was going to parcel up all the things that Leanne had sent him and send them back.

Leanne eventually cut all ties with Karl once she knew the truth. To her, I was the sick one. I was the one who had no one else and who was obsessed with Karl. You see, he was playing one off against the other. He could never tell anyone the truth, but would say what he thought the other person wanted to hear. He was doing the same thing with Sylvia. Karl was a master of spin and an expert in lies, and I only found out about the true extent of his double-dealings as time wore on. It was to be an education to me of how an illness can become all-pervasive in a person. Karl's illness took over both our lives.

After being in the mother and baby unit for 2 months, Karl was given a flat in Maida Vale. The grey cinder block was very depressing and soulless in a run down area, and the flat allocated to Karl was in a bad state of repair. It was dirty, had no carpets, precious few cupboards and was practically uninhabitable. In fact, it was the sort of place that features on BBC documentaries like 'Life of Grime'. It looked like someone had died there, or at least was about to. The view from the living room window overlooked a concrete playground, long since abandoned by children. It seemed that the only users were just that, users. If you looked closely, you could see groups of youths congregating around each other exchanging money for packages.

The few shops that served the area had bars and mesh on the windows, where they had been broken into time after time. The downstairs flats were similarly fitted out, including metal doors with more locks on them than the local bank. It was the kind of estate that the police would deem a 'no-go' area. We never saw any police patrolling the area.

Karl's parents had offered to carpet the place for him so that it was slightly more fit for human habitation and a friend of a friend had offered to carry out various repairs to the flat and put in a work surface for the kitchen. For my part, I did as best I could to help Karl clean the place, but it was very overwhelming as it was so filthy. We spent a fair amount of time shuttling back and forth between our flats trying to get his place habitable. As with most things, it seemed as if everyone was doing all the work and Karl did what ever he wanted. His mum and dad had paid for the carpets, his friend was working for practically nothing doing the repairs and I paid for various essentials, like cups and plates. What did Karl do? He bought a music system. He had no money for the essentials, like cleaning materials, but as soon as he got his benefit, he blew it on an expensive luxury. That was Karl all over, as I was to find out more and more as time wore on.

We decided that it would be a good idea if Karl could drive, as he could then get from his flat to my flat easier and we would be able to visit his parents more often. As Karl had no money and I had a few savings, I agreed to pay for his lessons. Meantime, Karl phoned his parents once or twice a week from my flat. During one of these phone calls, I overheard Karl's mum saying to him, 'You mustn't keep giving in to Sue. She can't keep having her own way. She's got to give a bit and move into your flat, not you all the time being in her flat.'

His parents wanted me to give up my flat and move in with him. Karl wanted it as well. I couldn't believe it. I was the stable one and I was the one financing things. If I had moved in with Karl, I would have been on skid row. When I told Mum and Dad about it, they were flabbergasted. They told me in no uncertain terms not to give my flat up. I didn't intend to. Not only did I hate the Maida Vale area, but also I had my job at Oakland's to consider, which I loved, and I was near my family, which I needed.

On the other hand, I was desperate for company and needed Karl in my life and loved having him in my flat. While he was there, I was more on an even keel. He didn't want to be on his own at the Maida Vale flat, so if he wasn't with me he was at his parent's house. He made every excuse, the flat wasn't ready, and he didn't have this thing or that thing. He also told his parents that I was preventing him from moving to the flat and that I wanted him to stay in my flat. Of course, there is a grain of truth in that. I found it hard to hold together on my own and that when Karl was there I could function better. However, I never said to him that I didn't want him to go back to his flat. Nevertheless, that's what he told his parents.

One day I received a phone call from Kay, and she said to me that Karl must be allowed to move into his flat and that I had to stop preventing him having his independence. I never stopped Karl from moving into his flat, but that is obviously what he told his mum. Once again, I was cited as the villain of the piece. Eventually, the flat was as ready as it was going to be. Karl had run out of excuses and moved into the flat.

As Karl was spending more and more time at my flat, we learned more and more about each other's problems. I knew about his 'mini' binges while he was at my flat, but he also explained about his big binges. During the day, he would consume no more than a cup of coffee, but each evening he would allow himself a cup of diet hot chocolate and a Chomp bar, which is a small chocolate covered toffee bar. Having said that, he never ate the bar but merely sucked off the chocolate and threw the rest away. If it was a 'good' day, that would be all he would have. Otherwise, he would have a mini binge in my flat. A mini binge would consist of a packet of biscuits, several chocolate bars and a couple of Chomp bars. None of these was consumed, but would be partly chewed and then spat out.

He would also rent a video to watch and a comic to read during this time. He did this all late at night once I had gone to bed. Karl and I didn't have a sexual relationship, so as I slept upstairs and he slept downstairs, it didn't affect me at all. If I had to come downstairs in the middle of the night to use the toilet, the light would still be on and there would be half spat out chocolate in paper towels and plastic bags. He never liked me to talk to him or acknowledge him if I caught him like this. He just wanted me out of the way so that he could carry on. It was an embarrassment for him, as if I had caught him with a dirty magazine or something. As I had a similar problem, in as much as I would binge eat out of unhappiness, I knew that it was a taboo area. If I challenged him too much he might decide not to stay with me.

When I came down the following morning, the dustbin would be full of packages of half-regurgitated food, and Karl would be dead to the world until at least lunchtime. Even though he didn't consume the majority of the food, he still felt bloated and stuffed, similar to how I felt when I had a binge, although in my case I had actually eaten the food. In that respect, I knew how he was feeling.

One night a week, however, he would have what he called a 'special time'. He used to go back to the Maida Vale flat for that. As the time approached for the special time, he would get into a heightened state of excitement. He would shop for everything he wanted for the evening. This was not just the food, he would also buy a special comic he wanted and he would hire a video that he wanted to watch. He would spend as much money as he had on what could be termed junk food. He would buy almost the entire stock of cakes from the local baker, plus chocolate bars and biscuits. Again, none of this was entirely eaten, but instead chewed and spat out.

After this binge, which carried on until the early hours of the morning, he would feel so awful about himself and so fat, that he would take a large quantity of sleeping pills washed down with cans of special brew. This combination obviously knocked him out cold, and he would be unconscious for most of the next day. The following day he would try to clean up the mess he had made and then make his way back to me, in a very distressed and depressed state. He would stay about three or four days before heading back to his flat to do it all again. He was as addicted to these sessions as an alcoholic would be to a drink or a gambler to a bet.

Julie and I were going to have a short break in Windsor, and we asked Karl if he would like to come with us. He had no money, but we said we would pay for him. The day before we were due to leave, I got a call from Karl saying that he was unable to go. His dad was going for tests at a hospital about his illness, and Karl wanted to be there for the results.

The day after Julie and I got to Windsor, I phoned Karl to hear the results. It was not good news. After x-rays and other tests, the hospital said that Tom had something wrong with his brain, that there was some shadow, but that they were not sure what it was. Karl told me that they would know more after they had done more tests, and that he would tell me the news when I got home.

After Julie and I got home from our break, I arranged to meet Karl for a concert at Kenwood. When I saw him, I could tell there was bad news. He was in a very distressed state, and when I asked him what was wrong he told me that the shadow on Tom's brain was a malignant brain tumour and that it was inoperable. He said that they were going to start chemotherapy and radiation treatment, and not to give up hope. Nevertheless, Karl was very down that day and naturally so was I. I liked Tom and hoped that he would get better. Needless to say, we didn't really enjoy the concert.

Karl carried on in earnest with his driving lessons, as it was now even more urgent to be able get to his parent's house. He passed his test first time, so obviously the next thing was to buy a car. With Julie's help, we went to look at various cars and we eventually bought a red mini metro. Karl's parents put up half the money and I put up the other half. At least, that's what I thought. I later found out from Kay that they had given Karl the whole amount of the car. He told me that they had only given half so that I would furnish him with the other half. He kept this money for his binge sessions.

This kind of deception would recur throughout our relationship. It wasn't that Karl wanted to steal from me. You see, like any compulsion it needed feeding. People who have compulsions are in a dilemma. On one hand, they hate themselves for what they have to do, be it gambling, eating, drugs etc, but paradoxically on the other hand they live for their obsessions and don't want them to stop. It sounds strange but it's true, believe me I know.

Because we now had a car, we were able to go and visit Karl's parents on a regular basis, and we could take them out or do a bit of shopping for them. Quite often during a visit, Karl would disappear upstairs to his room for periods, which left his mum, dad, and I alone. It was during these periods that I learnt more about Karl's binges. Tom and Kay told me that they went along with Karl's binges. In fact, Tom went along with him to the local bakers in a taxi and they more or less bought up the entire shop. Karl would tell the shopkeeper that he was a children's entertainer and he used the cakes for their parties.

Kay also baked on the day of the binge, and so all that was added to the food. Tom and Kay would then go to bed at night and leave Karl downstairs with a video that he had hired and his comics. He would set it all out like a tea party, with special paper plates and doilies and a roll of black bin sacks to spit the food into.

Karl had a nurse who would visit him after he came out of the Maudsley. When Tom and Kay told the nurse about Karl's binges without swallowing, he said that he must have been getting some nourishment inside him even if he didn't mean it. He suggested that they let him carry on as it was better than nothing.

The special needs department at Oakland's were looking for male volunteers, as they had very few. One of the head tutors, Barbara, knew of Karl and asked me if I would ask him if he would be interested. He agreed and started at Oakland's straight away. Well, he charmed everybody, as he always did. To give Karl his due, he was wonderfully kind, caring and patient with all the students he worked with. In that sense, he was well suited to the work. Barbara was completely enamoured with him, as were as all the other female staff and students.

Whereas I taught in the more formal classes, for example cookery, maths and assertiveness classes, Karl was more involved on the practical side. For example if we had to show the students how to buy a stamp from the post office or if we took the students on an outing to a garden centre or museum, Karl would help us in marshalling them. Of course, Karl still had his problems, but he worked at the college when he stayed with me, about three days a week. Then he would go back to his Maida Vale flat to have his 'special' times.

Meanwhile, my problems were the same as always. Although my eating was on a slightly more even keel when Karl stayed with me, for the rest of the time it was as bad as ever. I still had black depression and the fatigue was draining. Barbara used to give Karl and me a lift into college each morning, and I remember being so tired that I had to sit on the wall at the end of the road at Martins Court to wait for her car. I was so tired all the time that I could hardly walk. Whether it was the illness, the medication, the binge eating or a combination, I don't know. I was like a woman in her eighties. God knows how I managed to do a day at college.

WITNESS FOR THE PROSECUTION

Karl was offered part time paid work at Oakland's and because he hated his flat in Maida Vale, this was a good excuse to move out. He applied for a transfer to St. Albans and eventually got a flat in Abbotts Langley. This was good news for me, as it meant that he would be nearer. Barbara, the senior tutor of the Special Needs department, helped with the move and I did my best to sort the flat out once he was in. Karl settled into his flat, although it was only really used for his 'special times'. The rest of the time he stayed at my flat.

While Karl was working at Oakland's, he was offered a full time job at a new residential home in Wheathampstead, near St. Albans. This was a home for patients who couldn't fend for themselves. The job involved shift work, but that was all right, as he had a car to get him there. One day I was expecting him home but he was very late. When he eventually came in, he was very shaken up. He told me that he had been involved in a road accident. He said that another car came out of a side road and smashed into the side of him. He wasn't hurt, but the passenger side of the car was smashed in. He said that he had to leave the car in a side road, as it was un-drivable.

'Did you get the other drivers insurance details?' I asked

'No' he said, 'he wasn't insured'.

'Well then, you surely got his name and address' I asked, knowing what the answer was going to be.

'No', he said. 'He told me that he had no fixed abode and that he had been living with his sister in her caravan'.

He told me that the man had several kids and that he wouldn't be able to pay a fine. I personally think that Karl didn't challenge the man at all, as he never liked conflict of any sort. So I don't know what really happened. I only know that the car was a write off and as we only had third party insurance, that was that.

Without a car we were stuck. We couldn't visit Karl's parents and he would be unable to get to work. Although there was the occasional bus that ran from St. Albans to Wheathampstead, it was only on alternate Tuesdays with an 'R' in the month, or so it seemed anyway. He phoned his parents and told them of the predicament, but they told him that they couldn't afford to give him any more money for another car, so I had to pay for it. I begrudged paying out a lot of money, as I didn't have much. We eventually found a clapped out Ford Escort, so I bought that.

I later found out that in fact when Karl phoned his parents about the money for a car, they readily agreed. Once again he lied to me and kept the remaining money for himself. I must have been blind. But then, love is.

As Karl was staying in my flat more and more, subsequently the massive binges took place there rather than at his flat. They were much worse now than I had witnessed in the past. Unless you live with this problem first hand, you have no idea what's involved. He became so frenzied in his rituals that when I came down in the morning I would find food splattered all over the walls. There was spat out food over the furniture and rugs, and his bed sheets were also covered in half eaten food mixed with spittle. His hands would have been covered in chocolate, so that anything he touched would also be smeared with chocolate and cream cakes. If you have ever witnessed the mess a toddler can make eating a bar of chocolate, just multiply that ten fold. It was as disgusting as it sounds, and for someone like me who had a problem doing ordinary housework, it was a nightmare.

Because of this I was in a difficult situation. On the one hand I liked Karl being there as it helped with my food problem and I had company, but on the other hand I was feeling more and more out of control because my flat was in such a disgusting state.

Because Karl was spending every penny he had on his problem, he wasn't paying any bills. In fact, he never paid any bills. Once he was due to go to court for non-payment of poll tax and asked me for the money. He owed about £170. I was getting fed up with bailing him out and never being repaid. I wanted him to have a bit of responsibility and actually pay his way in life, so I asked my sister Julie if she would lend him the money. I thought that he wouldn't be so cavalier with her.

Julie, being the kind soul she is, promptly lent him the money and he paid the bill. He had no choice. It was either that or risk imprisonment. Mind you, he wasn't so fast at paying Julie back. I had to stand over him while he wrote out a cheque for her. He paid back £70, leaving around £100 outstanding. He cried his eyes out in front of Julie, and said that he couldn't afford the rest. Julie felt sorry for him and told him that he could forget the balance.

Julie told me that after she told him that, she caught him with a sly smile on his face. He had won again. For all I know, he may have even got the money from his parents as well. He was a regular con man. Once his parents gave him some money for Christmas to help with his bills, but instead of using it to pay off some of his debts, he went straight into a computer shop and bought a Play Station.

Once a fortnight we went to see Karl's parents. Karl's dad, Tom, was going through chemotherapy and radiotherapy and we thought that the treatment was working. The hospital said that the tumour was shrinking. We were living in hope, as you do.

While I was working at Oakland's, we had various volunteers that came to work for us. Some of these people had problems of their own, but Barbara was very kind hearted and would take them on. One of these people was a man called Chris. Chris was quite an attractive man and looked not unlike the actor Tommy Lee Jones.

To all intents and purposes he was a normal, healthy individual who only wanted to help. I watched him work and although he was competent enough, I didn't feel that this type of work suited him particularly. He didn't have enough patience with the clients, and although he never shouted at them and certainly never hit them, he wasn't overly sympathetic with them either. However, Barbara liked him and she found out that he was attracted to me. Barbara knew of my situation with Karl and thought that I could do better. Therefore, she tried to engineer it so that Chris and I would get together.

One day there was to be a birthday party at one of the student's homes. I thought that I was going in Barbara's car but she arranged for Chris to take me. He stayed quite close to me throughout the party, as he knew no one there, and then dropped me off home after.

A few days later in college, he asked me out for a drink. I said yes, because although I loved Karl, I was fed up with the way he was treating me with his lies and I hated the after affects of his binging. I was also quite flattered that an attractive man asked me out. I, the repulsive, ugly Susan Kennedy that the boys at school said shouldn't be touched with a barge pole.

However, as the time for the date grew nearer I reconsidered. I told Chris that I couldn't go out with him because although I was living a crap life with Karl, I felt that he needed me and despite all else, I still loved him. He seemed all right about it, and we left it at that. The fact that this man liked me and was attracted to me thrilled me no end. Although I knew that nothing would come of it, the very thought of someone 'normal' fancying me got me through the days.

A short while later I was offered a fridge from my friend Dana. She had dropped it off at Mum and Dad's house but I had no way of picking it up from there. Chris stepped in and offered, as he had access to a van. When we went round to pick it up, Dad took me to one side and said that he liked the look of him, and thought that it would be a good idea if I had him as a boyfriend instead of Karl. To be honest, my family were so against Karl that they would have thought Attila the Hun would be a better bet.

Back at the flat, Chris kept saying that he fancied me and that I would be better off without Karl. I could see that he was infatuated with me and I suppose I was flattered. Although I never encouraged him and I certainly wouldn't have abandon Karl for him, similarly I didn't discourage him. This went on for a while at work, but it all came to a head one evening while I was alone in my flat, as Karl was at work. There was a knock on my door. It was Chris. I could tell he had been drinking. He came in and started again on how I was perfect for him and that I should leave Karl, and before long had his arms around me and started kissing me. I have to admit that I responded. Although I loved Karl, we were just soul mates and there was never a physical side to our relationship. I was also still a virgin and inside I wanted to know what a proper relationship was like.

Chris gripped my arms so tight that I had bruises on them for days after. He pulled me down on the ground and his hands were all over me. I knew what he wanted and deep down I wanted it as well. However, something inside me told me that it was wrong. I was thrilled that someone wanted me and that the sight of me didn't make them feel sick, as that was my opinion of myself since school days. He started to undo his trousers, but I couldn't let him do it. I had to put a stop to this; it was getting out of control. I pushed him away and said that I didn't want to do it. He got up, but I could see that he was angry. Just as he was doing his flies up, Karl walked in. He demanded to know what was going on. Chris and I were obviously in a dishevelled state and rapidly tried to make ourselves look presentable. I mumbled that there was nothing going on, and Chris said something like he had just called round to see if the fridge was working all right. Karl obviously didn't believe us and I could see that he was hurt.

Before anything more could be said, there was a knock at the door. It was one of the neighbours. He said that two mentally handicapped people had got out of Karl's car and were wandering around the car park. Karl ran off to round them up. It seemed that he had a suspicion of what was going on and called round on his way to the residential home with two of his clients. If he had been caught, he would have been sacked, but I don't suppose that entered his head at the time.

Alone now with Chris, I was feeling pretty bad. I blamed myself for encouraging him, or at least not discouraging him. He looked at me and said, 'All right, I'll go now. But I'll be back. And when I do I want to have sex with you.'

With that he went. Really, I shouldn't have given someone like that houseroom. However, in my defence, at that time I was very sick and fed up with the life I was leading. I loved Karl, but it wasn't a proper relationship. I wanted someone who would look after me and take care of me. I didn't want a life of constantly bailing someone out of debt, of false tears, the lies, the deceits, the clearing up of the mess after the binges. I wanted a real relationship. Was that too much to ask? I was desperate for a life, but in my desperation, I was making things worse.

When I went back to college, I told Barbara what had happened. I used to tell her everything. It so happened that just around that time Chris had applied for a job at a care centre. He had been offered the job subject to references. Barbara had written him a good reference, but on hearing what I told her, had decided to write to the day centre with an updated reference. She didn't mention this to me, but she told them that she had noticed that Chris had a short temper with the clients. It was true that he did have a short fuse, as I had also witnessed it, although he was never violent with them.

Armed with this new information, the care home had withdrawn their offer of a job. Chris was livid, especially with me, as he thought that I had put Barbara up to writing the bad reference. I did tell Barbara what had happened, but I didn't even know that Chris had applied to work at a day centre, nor that Barbara had given him a reference. I certainly didn't know that she then rescinded it.

One day I was in my flat with Karl, when there was a knock at the door. I opened it, and to my horror saw that it was Chris. He pushed his way past me into the living room where Karl was. There was anger etched all over his face. He came up to me, face inches from mine, screaming that I had ruined his chances of a career and that he was going to give me my just deserts. I was terrified. I had no idea what he was talking about, and in a halting, petrified voice tried to tell him so.

At that point, Karl tried to protect me and got between Chris and me. He told Chris to leave me alone, that I had done nothing. This was just the excuse Chris needed to vent his fury. He screamed at Karl, 'All you do is bring grief. You're a disgrace. You have no business defending anyone'.

With that, he attacked Karl and laid into him like a mad man. He was punching and kicking him, while I tried in vain to separate them. In Karl's condition, he was unable to defend himself. He kept sobbing, 'Leave her alone, leave her alone' whilst being pummelled.

Karl ended up curled in a ball sobbing under the stairs. Chris then came up to me, looked me straight in the eyes and said in a menacing way, 'If you say anything about this to anyone, you're dead. Don't think you've heard the last of this. I'll be back for you and then I'll move on to Barbara. I'll work my way through the list of everyone who has ever got in my way'. He then stormed out of my flat and slammed the door.

I turned round to see the flat looking like a bombsite. The furniture was thrown everywhere and some of it was broken. My eyes then went to Karl. He looked in a dreadful state; bruised, bleeding, unable to move and obviously in a state of shock. He kept saying, 'I'll be all right, I'll be all right', but it was evident that he wasn't. Although he had many faults, one of his positive traits was that he was a gentle person. He had been bullied and tormented at school, as I was, but he never fought back. Like me, he was one of life's victims and just took it.

I phoned for an ambulance and they took us to Hemel Hempstead Hospital. On examining Karl, apart from the cuts and extensive bruising to his face and body, they said that he had three fractured ribs. That maniac Chris could have killed him. That reinforced his threat to me and that he was capable of anything.

Karl and I had no way of getting home, so I phoned Barbara. When Barbara arrived and saw the state of Karl, she naturally wanted to know what happened. When I told her about Chris threatening to kill me then go after her, she was stunned.

'You must tell the police', she said. 'Even if you're not worried about yourself, think about me. I'm a single mother with three children to consider. You have to tell the police and get that thug off the streets'.

I was not so sure. I didn't want trouble, I never have. I just wanted things to be back the way they were. Neither Karl nor I wanted police involvement. As the days wore on, Barbara phoned constantly trying to get me to contact the police and report Chris. Eventually I relented and Karl and I went to St. Albans police station. We made a statement and told the officer what had happened. I said to him that I blamed myself. I said that I should have told Chris in no uncertain terms that I wasn't interested in him physically and that would have prevented all this. The police officer said that I shouldn't blame myself. He said that I didn't deserve to have someone push his way into my home, beat up my partner, smash up my furniture and then have my life, and other lives, threatened.

'By the way,' asked the police officer, 'do you know where Chris lives?'

I gave him the address of the flat that Chris gave me and he went off to do some checking. When he came back, he said, 'That address you gave me. It's for a bail hostel. This Chris is known to the police.'

I was shocked. It certainly explained a lot. The police officer didn't go into any detail about why Chris was on bail, but it didn't look good for him. Similarly, it didn't look good for me, either. If Chris found out that I had reported him to the police for assault and it meant that he would possibly have to go to prison for it, he definitely would come looking for me. I felt that I had been left carrying the can for Barbara.

A few weeks later, there was a knock on the door of my flat. I had put a spy hole in by now, as I was frightened of Chris coming back. Through the spy hole, I could see a rather dishevelled girl standing there. I opened the door, and as I did so, I caught her quickly turn her head, as though she was looking at someone who was keeping out of sight. I found out later that the person keeping out of sight was Chris, and this was his girlfriend. She was dressed shabbily and had an old battered handbag, obviously to play on my sympathies. She asked me if I had been having an affair with Chris, so I just told her the truth. I blamed myself, as I always do. She begged me not to go ahead with the court case, as they had no money and didn't know what to do if Chris ended up in prison. I told her that it was out of my hands now, and besides, I had promised Barbara that I would go ahead with it. Chris couldn't go around breaking people's ribs and threatening their lives.

She went, but a few weeks later I saw her in town with her little boy. She was not the poor, shabbily dressed person that came to my flat. She had expensive clothes and shoes on and looked quite well off. They were both looking at me and laughing. I later found out that she was the manageress of a pub in Borhamwood, and Chris used to visit her whenever he was allowed out of the hostel. Obviously, I didn't know Chris was seeing this woman, as he told me he was alone. Once again, I had been conned by an expert.

Eventually the case came to court. There was no sign of Barbara, as indeed there hadn't been during the run up to it. She wanted nothing to do with the proceedings, even though the case had only been brought to court on her insistence. The trial was a horrible time for us. The police barrister was useless, all he kept doing was yawning throughout the proceedings. Chris's barrister, on the other hand, was as good as money could buy. He didn't put Chris on the stand, probably because he knew that he was as guilty as sin. Karl and I had to take the stand though, and he put us through hell. He even brought up Karl's anorexia, as if that had anything to do with it. During the whole trial, Chris stared hatefully into my eyes. If looks could kill, the charge would have been murder.

Chris's barrister said that I was a femme fatale. I didn't really know what that meant. When I got home I looked it up. The dictionary described it as 'an unscrupulous woman who seduces or exploits men'. Seduces or exploits men? Me? I was the one being exploited. Despite Chris's barrister blaming everyone but his client, (as I suppose defence lawyers do), he was found guilty. We never found out what sentence he received though, because the judge said that there were other charges that he had to answer, unrelated to our case. It became clear that Chris was quite a villain, hence his stay in a bail hostel. It seems that he was no stranger to prison.

The anticlimax to this story is that we never knew what happened to Chris after that, and I never saw him again. I told Barbara the outcome of the trial, but she seemed indifferent to it. I felt used. After all, Barbara wanted the thing to go to court in the first place, because she was scared for her own safety. What about me? I had been instrumental in helping the police possibly putting someone in prison. What if Chris sought revenge? It would be me he would go after, not Barbara.

KARL HAS DAYS TO LIVE

One morning I was woken by a phone call from the home in Wheathampstead where Karl worked. He hadn't arrived. To all intents and purposes he'd gone, but I didn't see him go as I slept upstairs and he slept down. He had been due to start at 6:00 a.m. and it was now past seven. I was very worried, as Karl had to take sleeping pills to get off to sleep at night and he also drank strong beer, plus he took other medication, so he wasn't really fit to drive a car at that time of the day or at any time of the day.

Soon after, I got another call, and it was Karl. He was in a very distressed state, and told me that he'd had an accident. He said that someone had run into him and that he was all right but he would be late for work. He asked me to phone the home and explain. I duly phoned the home and spoke to a girl called Liz. I told her what had happened to Karl, and she said, 'What again?'

I asked her what she meant and she said that it had happened before. She said that a number of times Karl had been late for work and said that someone had run into him.

Well, this was news to me. She said, 'To be honest Sue, I wonder if Karl should be driving at all. I wonder if people really have run into him or has it been him running into things'.

It transpired that the wheel rims were all buckled, which is often caused by hitting a curb rather than another vehicle hitting you. I might have known that he would lie about that, just as he lied about everything else. Quite soon after that, the personnel manager asked to see Karl. She was obviously worried about him as she had heard about his numerous car accidents and his subsequent late arrivals. However, apart from that, his weight had dropped dramatically. He was now in a worse state than many of the clients in the home. The personnel manager suggested that he had some time off, in order to do something about himself. Although it was a suggestion, he obviously had no choice.

By this time, he had given up his flat in Abbotts Langley. I was quite happy for Karl to give up his flat, as my illness was getting no better and I needed someone there all the time, in order for me to cope. However, the news didn't go down too well with my mum and dad, and they decided to cut me off. They said that they would have nothing more to do with me while I had Karl in my flat. They thought that it was doing me more harm than good, which in hindsight it almost certainly was.

I did see Julie from time to time, although she had to come round without Mum and Dad knowing, as they had forbidden her to have anything to do with me. Being cut off from my parents was very hard for me. I was, and still am, very close to them, especially my mum. I used to look forward to having Sunday dinner with them and occasionally a phone call. They never came round my flat once Karl came on the scene. I was also very ill myself and I was unable to cope with housework, so Mum used to do my washing and ironing. I now had that to do, on top of Karl's washing and ironing. When you add Karl's problems to the equation, the binges and the mess that went with them, you can imagine my predicament.

But what could I do? I had to do what I thought was best for me to be able to survive. That meant having Karl with me. Also, rightly or wrongly, I loved him very much. He was very needy and I couldn't abandon him.

Occasionally, one of the girls from the Wheathampstead home would come to Oakland's to drop clients off. I knew all the girls fancied Karl, as he was very charming, and with his blond hair and blue eyes, it's easy to see why. If any of them saw me, they would tell me that I should be kinder to Karl and not give him such a rough time. They said similar things if ever I went to the Wheathampstead home. Obviously, Karl was maligning me to these girls and telling them that I was the cause of all his problems. Once again, I was the villain of the piece.

Things were deteriorating rapidly for Karl. He was getting more and more depressed, the weight was dropping off him rapidly, and his binges and food obsession was all-encompassing. With what little strength he had, he would go to the local garage to get chocolate and cakes, which he would look at, feel, chew and spit out.

I used to go regularly to see my GP, Dr. Gorton. He knew all about Karl, as he was also his GP now. One day, while I was there, I broke down in his surgery and told him what was going on. He said, 'You shouldn't be going through this on your own. You need help. In addition, the weight Karl is now is very dangerous. He could die at any time'.

Although Karl had begged me not to call a doctor in to him, I felt that I had no choice. It was either that or watch him die in my flat. When Dr. Gorton saw Karl lying in bed, he was aghast. It was a while since he had seen him and he was shocked at how much weight he had lost. Dr. Gorton said that Karl would have to go to Hill End, which was a general psychiatric Hospital. Karl begged him not to send him there. Dr. Gorton said that he would try to get Karl into an eating disorder clinic, but in the meantime, he would have to go to Hill End, right now, just to save his life.

Karl kept beseeching me to let him stay in the flat for one more night. Dr. Gorton said that Karl might not have one more night left. He looked at me and said that if I were to allow Karl to stay there even for one night, the responsibility would be mine, and if Karl died as a result, it would be on my own conscience. He said that I would have to sign a form to the effect that if Karl died, it would not be down to medical negligence but my own choice. He added that if Karl didn't go in by the next day he would have no choice but to section him.

I was in a dilemma, but what could I do? I wanted Karl to go into hospital to get better, but I didn't want to force him into it. As I was showing Dr. Gorton to the door, he turned and winked at me. He said that he wasn't going to let me shoulder all the responsibility for Karl, but he wanted to frighten him into going into hospital. After Dr. Gorton left, Karl promised me that he would go into hospital of his own accord, as long as he could have one more binge. I agreed, and the next day Karl went in to Hill End.

Hill End Hospital was an old Victorian mental hospital, and quite close to my flat in St. Albans. It doesn't exist any more as it was closed and knocked down like so many other mental hospitals up and down the country. As we walked down the long, dingy corridors, I had a feeling of déjà vu. It was the Maudsley all over again. I was expecting the same uninterested and miserable ward orderlies to meet us. I was pleasantly surprised when a dark haired, rather attractive man came up to us and introduced himself as Les. Les told us that he ran the ward that Karl was to be on. He came across as extremely caring and compassionate, towards me as well as Karl. In my experience, it was very rare to find someone like that in a mental hospital. The few good ones stand out like a beacon on a stormy night; Hilary from the Maudsley and of course, David Britten from the Gordon Hospital. Most of the others, however, were there because they either couldn't speak English and couldn't get another job or else they were just bone idle, and they could do as much or as little as they wanted. The vast majority of them were either cruel and sadistic or lazy and apathetic and more often, a combination of those characteristics, which is why the few dedicated ones stick in your mind.

There were two single rooms on the ward. A man with bipolar disorder, otherwise known as manic depression, occupied one and Karl was allocated the other. The general ward had a mixture of patients suffering from various illnesses. One such patient was a man who wanted to become a woman. This man was well known in St. Albans and in fact, I had dealings with him myself during my time at the Abbey National Building Society. He changed his name like other people changed their socks. While he was in Hill End, he was so high on drugs he was almost hanging from the ceiling.

There were also a number of alcoholics on the ward, who would go out during the day and get drunk then come back later on and smash the ward up. Hill End didn't really know how to deal with eating disorders, and really, it was used as a holding area until a place at an eating disorder clinic became available.

The problem with Karl was that he had been a patient at various eating disorder hospitals, for example the Maudsley and the Gordon. The experts had recognised that his problems were bigger than first thought. They knew that he needed expert help to survive so it was essential that he went to a specialised unit. The trouble was that these places were at a premium and cost the earth to run. Karl's track record of using and abusing the system was well known, therefore no hospital manager was prepared to risk his budget on someone who was not 100% committed to beating the problem. It's a bit like an alcoholic or drug addict being given the chance to go to a unit to overcome their problem. If they then abuse the system, then they get no second chance. There are just too many people on the waiting list. As a result, Karl remained in Hill End for quite a while.

Karl had his car parked at Hill End, and every day when the staffs' backs were turned, he would drive to the local garage to stock up on cakes and chocolates, which he then smuggled back into his room to binge on. Of course, all this food cost money. Although I brought him in pocket money each day for cigarettes, he spent much more than his allowance. He got around this by telling me that he had his money stolen. I knew it was true that other patients had had their money stolen, as there were a number of rogues on the ward who would take whatever they could lay their hands on. Therefore, when Karl told me that it had happened to him, I readily agreed to give him some more.

This happened on a number of occasions, and finally I decided to challenge Les about it. However, when I confronted Les about Karl's missing money he didn't seem overly worried, and in fact dismissed it. I found this strange, as he was usually a very caring person. On hindsight, I realise that Les must have known what was going on but couldn't prove it. Once again, I was the last to know that I was being conned by Karl.

Les was quite an incisive man. He watched me day after day coming in and caring for Karl, and he could see the effect it was having on me. One day he called me in his office for a chat. He said that he was worried about me and that I had to start thinking of myself, as well as Karl, as he could see that I was going down hill rapidly. He said that I had to be hard, think of number one for a change and leave Karl to get on with it. He said that if I didn't, then I would go under.

Of course, I couldn't do that. I could never abandon Karl, even though I knew what was happening to my health. Les understood and said that whatever happened, he would help me in any way that he could. He said that his wife had been anorexic and through their love for each other, she had managed to beat the illness. In fact, she was expecting a baby. That made me more determined to stick by Karl. I thought in my naïveté that I could cure Karl through love. I couldn't have been more wrong.

Although Karl had his binge sessions, little of the food managed to enter his stomach, with the result that Karl was losing weight rapidly. In order to induce Karl to eat something, Les used psychology on him. He pointed out to Karl that there were a number of patients on the ward, alcoholics, drug addicts and the like, who were losing their respective partners. The wives or girl friends just couldn't take it any more. Les told Karl that he was very lucky to have me, but that if he carried on losing weight and refusing to eat, I would stop visiting him. He told Karl that he was going to phone me each day, and if he told me that Karl had eaten, then I would visit. On the other hand, if Karl refused to eat anything then he would report that to me and I would stay away.

I don't really know what happened to that system, as I phoned Les every day to see if Karl had eaten and he regularly said yes. However, when I visited Karl I could see that he was getting thinner and thinner. I expect that Les didn't want me to stop visiting Karl, as I was his last hope.

Karl became so thin and weak that he wasn't physically able to wash himself or to shave. The ward orderlies told me that it wasn't in their job description to wash Karl, so I would have to do it. I would have liked to see their job description. It must have said something like sitting about all day watching television and drinking tea. I agreed to do it and subsequently went in each day to bathe Karl, shave him and anything else that was necessary. Bearing in mind that with my illness I had enough trouble bathing myself, this was no mean feat.

At the same time that Karl was in Hill End, Tom's cancer was getting progressively worse. The doctors told Kay that it was just a matter of time now. They said that he possibly had three months to live. A Macmillan nurse came in regularly to tend to Tom, as he refused to go into hospital. Obviously, Karl's dad was too ill to visit Karl, and his mum was too busy looking after Tom to visit herself. However, Karl and Kay used to phone each other quite regularly. After a while, however, Karl became so weak that he didn't have the strength to walk to the pay phone. During that time, I used to field the calls between them. I tried to spare Karl the increasingly depressing news of Tom's illness and at the same time, I was trying to spare Kay and Tom the pain of Karl's worsening condition.

I was the piggy in the middle, trying to keep both sides' happy, keeping things afloat and trying not to sink without trace myself. I was desperately ill, and trying to cope with terminal illnesses was not helping. What I had to contend with would be hard for someone who was fit and well. I was far from fit and well.

As Karl was ostensibly at deaths door, he was on ‘open order’. That meant that he could have visitors at any time. He didn’t want visitors apart from me, but Julie would come on occasion. Those visits were a nightmare. She would turn up unannounced, armed with religious relics and prayer books, and attempt to hold her own mini service. She meant well, but she was mentally ill herself, and she went on and on and on about what he should do and why he should eat and if he held this religious relic or said that prayer he would get better. Karl wasn’t going to eat no matter what Julie, or anyone else, said. He didn’t have the strength to fight her and neither did I. Nevertheless, she went on regardless. She was manic and irrational and didn’t help matters at all. Julie was obsessed with her religion and believed it was a cure all. I’m afraid it wasn’t and isn’t. Julie was trying to help, but in reality, was making matters worse.

Before I lost my job at Oakland’s, and was essentially on compassionate leave, Barbara also used to visit Karl occasionally. I still regarded her as a friend at that time, and indeed, she behaved like one. She even took Karl to see his dad one day, as there was no way I could get him there.

One day Karl had an unexpected visitor. Her name was Molly and she was the head of the Wheathampstead home where Karl worked. She was a motherly, caring type, and was supportive of Karl and of me. As with the ward manager Les,

Molly was someone that I leaned on heavily, someone that Karl and I respected, and we regarded her as our ally and our friend. She started visiting often and both Karl and I appreciated her concern.

Molly suddenly stopped visiting Karl, which seemed very strange. When I next saw Barbara, I asked her if she knew if Molly was ill, as it seemed so out of character for her to stop visiting. Barbara told us that we wouldn't be seeing Molly again as she was on the run from the police. I couldn't believe what I was hearing. Apparently, Molly and her husband, who was a chef, had run up debts of thousands of pounds. As head of the home, she was responsible for all the finances and had access to both the patients' money and the home's money. She had embezzled thousands of pounds and had now vanished without trace with all the money.

To say that I was shocked would be an understatement. You think you know someone then you get a bombshell like that. I always speak as I find, and Molly was always a good friend to both Karl and I. We trusted her and she was supportive of us, but obviously, there was another side to her.

While Karl was in Hill End, there was a new eating disorder clinic under construction, called the Peter Dally clinic, which was part of the Westminster Hospital. This was to be run by none other than David Britten, who ran the eating disorder clinic in the Gordon Hospital. I rang David, whom I considered a friend, as he had been supportive of both Karl and me. I wanted to see if I could get

Karl into his new clinic, as I knew that Hill End was doing no good for him. However, David was reluctant to take Karl. He said that he was fund manager as well as director of the unit, and had to justify every penny he spent. He said that it was terribly costly treating patients and therefore they only took the ones they thought would benefit. He said that he couldn't afford to take anyone who would be likely to abuse the system. He knew Karl, and thought that he would certainly abuse the system.

The next day, when I went to visit Karl, one of the doctors took me aside to speak to me. He told me that Karl was dying. He said that he had days, rather than weeks to live. He told me what signs to look out for and he said that there would be a crash team on standby. Of course, I was devastated. When I got home in the evening, I phoned everywhere, begging them to take Karl in. But of course, it was just little me fighting the system. You can't just ring a hospital and say, 'Please can you take my boy friend in?'

You have to have financing from your local authority, and they were not prepared to finance Karl, as they believed that he didn't want to get well. They thought, quite rightly probably, that he wouldn't work with the treatment that he had to have. I asked Les for his help. As he knew many of the legal and medical loopholes, and some high up management, Les eventually managed to get Karl a place in the Bethlem Royal Hospital in Beckenham, Kent. The Bethlem is the sister hospital of the Maudsley, and is also where the name 'bedlam' comes from, which is quite apt.

The next day, an ambulance came for Karl to take him to the Bethlem. They had to drive painfully slowly, as he had bedsores, ruptures and abrasions all over his body, as he was just bones. I didn't go with him, as it was too early in the morning. However, I went in to his room at Hill End to clear it out. It was as I was clearing it out that I found all the food concealed in the drawers and hidden behind the wardrobe. It hit home then just how sick he was and how much a prisoner of his illness he had become. The discovery of the food was not a surprise for Les. He had a suspicion of what had been happening, which is why he didn't show much concern about the robberies that Karl had alleged happened.

THE BETHLEM

The Bethlem Hospital is set in magnificent grounds, surrounded by beautiful countryside. A long, tree lined drive sweeps up to the old Victorian buildings. You could be mistaken for thinking that it was a country mansion of one of the nobility if you didn't know that it was a mental hospital. However, the inside was far from beautiful. It was stark, bleak and as depressing as the Maudsley and Hill End.

When Karl arrived at the Bethlem, he insisted that he walked from the ambulance to the ward. I don't know how he did it, as he was so weak and near death's door. One of the nurses told me that she had never seen willpower like it. It was just a pity that it was never used in a more positive way.

The most horrible, black nurse I had ever seen ran the eating disorder ward. I have come across quite a few sadistic and cruel nurses and orderlies in my time, but she outshone them all. She had not one ounce of compassion or feeling in her body. I can't remember her name, but she was as round as she was tall. She waddled around with a big bunch of keys hanging from her waist, and looked as if she had materialised from the original Bedlam Hospital. Whilst it was true that the patients in her charge had to follow a strict regime, she made sure they suffered as a result. She also treated me and other visitors in the same, sneering, insensitive way. She always seemed to be there, hanging around in the background. The first time that I visited Karl I had to see him in a corridor. She wouldn't allow visitors in patient's rooms and she wouldn't provide a room for visitors to meet patients. That wasn't hospital policy you understand, that was just her.

My enduring memory is seeing Karl looking like a stick insect, clinging to the bars that ran the length of the corridor to come and meet me. The state he was in, (he could hardly stand), one would have thought that a chair at least would have been a good idea. Although there were annexes and rooms we could have used, she wouldn't allow it. Bitch!

She also had the habit of hovering around us, so that she could eavesdrop on our conversation. After about 15 minutes, she would call a halt to my visit and make me leave. When you consider that it took me 3 hours to get there and another 3 hours to get home, to only allow me 15 minutes was cruel. It was as if the people in her care were not patients, but murderers on death row. In fact, I wouldn't mind betting that murderers on death row get better treatment.

Naturally, Karl was very unhappy. The regime he had to live with made him more and more depressed, and along with all the other patients, he had his remaining dignity taken away. He was only allowed one phone call a week, which would have been bad enough in normal circumstances, but he obviously wanted to keep in touch with his mum for any news about his dad.

As with the Maudsley, when patients went to the toilet, they had to leave the door open. If they didn't, this nurse would kick the door open, stand there with her arms folded, and watch. I know she did this, as she did it with me once when

I used the toilet. She thought that I was a patient. Of course, I got no word of apology from her. Mind you, she was completely different with the visitors of the private patients. She was all smiles with them and they got a private room to visit their sons or daughters. The rest of us had to lump it. I know life isn't fair, but if I had a genie in a bottle, I would wish that sadistic and heartless lowlife like her, would get an illness and have to suffer the same treatment that she dished out.
During this time Tom's illness had progressed to such a degree that he had to move in to a hospice. The hospice was in Maida Vale, coincidentally near to Karl's old flat. I told Kay that I would go and stay with her for a week, because she found it hard to cope on her own. She was all right when she had Tom around, even though he was desperately ill. Just his being there gave her the strength to carry on. Because Kay suffered from agoraphobia she couldn't go out on her own, so I accompanied her to and from the hospice by train. I used to see how Tom was and then I left them to be on their own while I went for a walk around the Maida Vale area.

The hospice was lovely. There were many bright colours, and it seemed like an upmarket nursing home. The staff were very nice and made Tom and all the other patients as well as visitors, as comfortable as possible. I have every admiration for them.

What a contrast between Tom's treatment and his son's. There you have two people with terminal illnesses, (or at least possibly terminal in Karl's case), treated by people from both ends of the spectrum. I was happy that Tom was in comfortable surroundings and getting the best of care.

Despite the gravity of the cases in the hospice, the place wasn't all doom and gloom. The doctors, nurses, or patients rarely talked about death or dying, and in fact, many of the conversations were of trivia; what's happening in Coronation Street, or plans for Christmas. I suppose people bury their heads in the sand. Having said that, if something is inevitable, why dwell on it. Make the most of the time you have available. Towards the end of their time, the patients are on stronger and more powerful drugs, so to some extent they're unaware of their surroundings in the closing stages. The doctors and nurses do their utmost to make the end as peaceful and dignified as possible.

Kay and I both knew that the end was near for Tom, and although the doctors told him, I don't think he took it in. Whether the brain tumour affected his thought patterns or whether he just blocked out the news himself, he seemed oblivious to the fact. He just carried on being his cheerful self, albeit getting weaker by the day. He would get emotional from time to time and cry, and petty things would upset him, like he didn't have any paper hankies or the orange juice wasn't right. Like my dad, Tom suffered from OCPD, (obsessive-compulsive personality disorder). I therefore understood why he got upset over trivia. As his world got smaller and smaller, he would concentrate on what we would consider insignificancies.

Karl knew that his father was in a hospice, although it didn't seem to affect him that much. I know that he was close to his dad, but perhaps his coolness was due in no small part to his own illness. Maybe he was so entrenched and so absorbed with his own illness that he didn't have any spare capacity to worry about anybody else. It's true that one of the consequences of eating disorders, especially Anorexia, is that feelings are stifled. The anorexic finds it hard to think beyond the illness. Of course, I couldn't know what Karl was going through inside or what he was feeling, but certainly to all intents and purposes, outwardly he seemed to accept what was happening to his father without much emotion. Indeed, it seemed like I was taking Tom's illness and impending demise much worse than Karl was. Of course, I was shouldering a lot of the strain. Karl had very little to do with what Tom and Kay were going through. He wasn't allowed out and he was only allowed one phone call a week and relied on me to relay any news.

As Tom's life was ending, he decided that he wanted to come out of the hospice and go home. They granted his wish, and an ambulance took him to his house. He obviously needed round the clock nursing care, which he got from the Macmillan nurses. I have a lot of time for these wonderful people. They do a lot of good to help not only people suffering from cancer, but just as importantly, the family and friends of the patients. Douglas Macmillan, who watched his own father suffer from cancer, set up the charity in 1911. Douglas wanted to make a difference to the care cancer patients received. There are now over 2500 Macmillan nurses in the UK, and I think Douglas Macmillan would be proud of each one of them.

I tried to do my best for Kay and help her as much as I could, and I visited Karl as often as I was able. I was finding it harder and harder to cope in my flat on my own, and the strain of it all took its toll on my Achilles heel, my eating. It was right off the wall. I didn't know who I could turn to for help. Mum and Dad had cut me off, and although I saw Julie, she wasn't well herself. I decided that I would contact Les from Hill End. I remember the story he told me of how his wife had beaten Anorexia, and I thought that maybe he would have the answer for me.

Les was quite an extrovert character, and of an evening, he would draw the patients around him and hold an impromptu quiz or game of charades. While Karl was a patient at Hill End, Les included me in these events, and I used to love them. These evenings were my social life; such was my sad life at the time.

Les told me to come to the hospital at the end of his shift, and he would see me. When I arrived on the ward, he took me into a side room and I poured out all my troubles to him. Obviously, he was already au fait with most of what I told him, but nevertheless, took the time to hear me out and was very sympathetic to me. People kept knocking on the door while we were having this discussion, so Les said to me, 'What are you like at making tea?'

'Not bad.' I replied.

'Good,' he said, 'then you meet me out by the gate, I'll give you a lift home on my motor bike, and you can make me tea.'

In hindsight, I realise that once again I was being naïve. Les was a caring person, but he didn't just want to be a shoulder to cry on. It would have been plain to anyone else that Les fancied me, but I just couldn't see it. Why should I? Wasn't I repulsive to the male population? Les took me back to my flat on the back of his bike, which was quite exciting for me, and I duly made him that cup of tea. I was very flattered that a man as nice and as caring as Les wanted to talk to me. Of course, he didn't want to talk.

Les sat on the sofa, while I sat on a chair facing him, waiting for the pearls of wisdom to pour forth from his lips. What he actually said was, 'What are you doing sitting over there? Come here and sit next to me.'

Over I went, and sat next to him, ready to continue our discussion, when in fact he drew me to him and started kissing me. I responded as I was flattered by the attention. Here was a man who had an element of power and who I looked up to. He was someone who I thought would never give the likes of me a second look. He suggested that we went upstairs, and to this day I don't know why I did, but I agreed. Obviously, he was awakening things in me that I didn't even know I had. Before I knew what was happening, our clothes were off and he got me into bed.

I then froze, as my inner self was telling me that this was wrong. I said to him, 'Please stop. I'm a virgin and I don't have any protection and I'm frightened.'

He stopped, looked at me and said, 'All right then. But I want you to know what a real man feels like. I want you to know what you could have, that you can't have with Karl.'

He then took my hand, put it on his erect penis, and got me to stroke it. Even while it was going on, I knew that it was wrong, but I was powerless to stop. I thought that it was nice of him not to have sex with me. Of course, that would have been rape, but I wasn't thinking straight. Once again, I blamed myself. It was my fault. I must have led him on. I thought that he was being a gentleman by constraining himself and being content with me doing this to him, despite the fact that he was getting all the pleasure out of it.

I thought of myself as a piece of worthless shit. He said that I had his phone number if I needed him again, as if I would. He put on his biker gear and left. I felt absolutely awful and sick. You see, I was desperate for company, for anyone who was going to stop the hell I descended into whenever I was alone, even if it meant that I acted like a prostitute. How could I degrade myself like that? Once again, I turned to the food, hating the very being that I was.

Just to finish this episode, I later found out from one of the orderlies on Les's ward, that Les's wife was giving birth around the time he was at my flat. Obviously, he was just using me as a stopgap whilst his wife was out of action, so to speak. That made me feel even worse. Of course, I knew he was married, but I didn't want an affair with him. However, to know that I did what I did while his wife was in labour made me want to throw up. Bastard!

Karl knew that his dad had just a few days to live and so asked for a leave of absence from the hospital in order to see him one last time. He was refused. It really was like serving a prison sentence. He appealed against this decision, and the hospital reluctantly allowed an orderly to accompany Karl to see his father for one hour. Understandably, this wasn't enough for Karl. How could it be? Karl phoned me and asked if I could get him out so that he could stay with his dad until the end. However, I was powerless. Karl had been sectioned and would not be released out of The Bethlem until the doctors sanctioned it.

That was not going to put Karl off, however. He escaped! The first I heard of it was when I got a phone call from Lynn, one of the nurses at the Bethlem. She said that Karl had escaped and she believed that he would make his way to my flat. She said that as his weight had gone up to around nine stone and his life was no longer in danger, the hospital would release him, provided he had somewhere to stay. The decision was mine, whether or not he could stay in my flat. Lynn said that the hospital's advice was for me to refuse to admit Karl to my flat, so that he would have nowhere to go and would be forced to complete his hospital treatment. This would not include being able to spend any more time with his dad.

What could I do? I knew that if it was my mum or dad, I would want to see them if they were dying. Before I knew it, there was a loud banging on my door. It was Karl. He was crying like a baby, begging me through the letterbox to let him in. Of course, I had to let him in. Despite everything, I still loved him, cared about him, and knew the pain he was going through.

As it turned out, Tom had a week left to live. Karl and I went down to Acton to see him several times that week, although for the most part he was unconscious from the morphine, and didn't know we were there. Tom died on December 4th, 1995. Karl wasn't there at the time, and I was glad that he wasn't. The Macmillan nurse had told Karl that Tom died peacefully in his sleep. That wasn't the case, however. Tom didn't believe in an afterlife and had fought right to the end; to save himself from the nothingness that he was sure was to follow. Kay told me that the last hour or two were pretty horrendous, with Tom struggling in agony fighting the inevitable.

The nurse had laid Tom out in the front room, and I accompanied Karl to pay our respects. He looked asleep and very peaceful. The nurse had propped a book up under his chin, to keep his mouth closed. The book was very poignant as Tom loved reading, and in fact, Kay had a wreath made in the shape of a book for the funeral.

Kay, quite naturally, was in a state of shock and was unable to organise anything, so I was quite glad to see that a number of relatives had turned up who could cope. Tom's identical twin had turned up, which was quite eerie, and Tom's sister. It was her husband, Karl's uncle, who took control of everything and arranged the funeral.

Karl and I stayed with Kay in the period leading up to the funeral. Not that we did much, as

Karl's uncle did the practical things, but I think that Kay appreciated the company. It wasn't easy for me. I found it hard to cope with ordinary everyday life, but here I was trying to cope with the most horrendous things. Instead of me relying on people to get me through the day, here I was, having to be strong.

We had about 4 days to go before the funeral, and I felt stifled just sitting in Kay's living room. There was nothing to do, so I suggested that we all went to Brent Cross for the day, just to get out of the flat. Kay didn't want to go but insisted that Karl and I went. When Kay went out of the room, Karl said to me, 'I don't want to leave Mum alone.'

I said, 'Look, we can't just sit here for 4 days doing nothing. We've offered our help, but she said that she doesn't want anything done. She doesn't want us to sort out Tom's clothes, which is understandable. I would really like her to come with us, but if she doesn't, we should go on our own. We're just sitting here twiddling our thumbs. It will do us good.' I added, 'At the end of the day, your mum's got to get on with her life on her own eventually.'

What I didn't realise at the time was that Kay was standing the other side of the door while I said all this. She took it completely the wrong way, to the effect that I didn't care about her, which was not true. I just wanted a break. Nevertheless, she held that against me for the rest of the time that I knew her, and she constantly threw it back at me. Despite all that I had done for her, supporting her while Tom was in the hospice, and after he died, those innocent words, taken out of content, ruined everything.

Karl and I did go to Brent Cross and we had an awful time. There were Christmas trees and lights, carol singers and happy smiling people doing their shopping, but Karl and I felt anything but festive, as you can imagine. I wished at the time that we hadn't gone.

KARL SECTIONED FOR CHRISTMAS

Karl and I had to go to the Bethlem to attend the official discharge meeting. He was back at my flat but was still nowhere near the weight he should have been and was still very ill. When we arrived, the head social worker and his assistant from St. Albans were there to meet us. Apparently, the Bethlem had contacted St. Albans social services because they felt that Karl was extremely vulnerable. They couldn't section him, but at the same time, they were worried about discharging him. I think that they were just covering their own backs.

We went into the meeting, and chairing the committee was Lynn, who had been a nurse at the Maudsley while I was there. She wasn't much good while she was at the Maudsley, and she was precious little good here. All this Lynn kept saying was, 'We want to be sure that we're covered. We want to be sure that it's not going to backfire on us.' She was only interested in looking after the Bethlem's reputation. She wasn't the least bit interested in Karl and his welfare.

After listening to this, the head social worker from St. Albans intervened and said, 'Do you have no compassion at all for the couple who are sitting here? All you're interested in is making sure that your own arses are covered.'

She replied, 'Look, I want to make sure there are no legal loopholes. We can't be held responsible for anything that happens to him once he leaves here.'

To which the social worker answered, 'Yes, well we're talking about people here.' He then turned to Karl and me and said, 'When this is all over, I would like you both to come and see me in my office in St. Albans.'

The hospital duly completed their requisite forms and discharged Karl, and we both left. On the way back home, we stopped at a Pizza Hut. I had already talked to him about how things had to change if he were to continue living in my flat. I said that if he were serious about beating the problem, then I would help him, as I tried to help him in a thousand different ways, a thousand times before. However, he would have to work with me. I said to him, 'All I'm asking you to do Karl, is to have a serve yourself salad in this Pizza restaurant. It's now dinner time and you've got to eat something.'

He wouldn't even do that for me. He got a couple of lettuce leaves and moved them around his plate for a while, but he refused to eat anything. We spent about three hours in this Pizza Hut, with me trying against all the odds to make Karl see sense. I only wanted him to help himself, but I was wasting my breath. Karl would promise you the world, but wouldn't change a thing. He couldn't. His illness was in charge.

A few days later, Karl and I duly went along to Edinburgh House in St. Albans, for our meeting with the chief social worker. Also at the meeting was a middle-aged woman called Mavis. As the meeting progressed, discussing what support Karl should get, Mavis looked at me and said, 'Well, we've discussed Karl. But who's supporting you?'

I said, 'Oh, I'm all right. I'm only here to support Karl and get him some help.'

Mavis said, 'Well, it seems to me that you've got a catalogue of problems yourself. You're trying to support, keep and help Karl in every way, with a ball and chain around your ankles. You have no support yourself. Even your own family have deserted you.' She went on, 'Whatever support Karl gets, I want to look after you, to make sure that you survive. I want to be your social worker.'

So there I was, with my very own social worker. I don't know what hoops Mavis had to go through to get me on her list, but from then on, I met up with her and had the backing and support of social services. Karl and I also had the continued support of Dr. Gorton. Although he didn't have any answers to our respective problems, he was a lovely man and a good listener. You could tell that he was rooting for us with our struggles against all the odds.

A few days before Christmas, Karl said that he wanted to go up to London to see his friend Ray, who lived in Maida Vale. I had met Ray a few times, and I liked him. He lived in a flat with his father and his mentally handicapped brother. Karl also wanted to sort out a few things for his mum. Before he died, Tom said that he wanted Kay settled. He didn't want her to stay in the rented house in Acton, that had a leaking roof, an exorbitant rent, and a landlord who did nothing. Therefore, they agreed together that Kay would move into a warden controlled flat in Swindon,

Wiltshire. To that end, she put her name on the waiting list, so that she could move as soon as possible. As luck would have it, a flat became available the following January. Kay's sister, who lived in Wiltshire, came up to London to help her pack and to move her to her new home.

I was glad that Karl wanted to go to London for a few days. I was at the end of my tether with him now. He'd had so many chances and had blown them all. He'd also had so much money off me that I had no chance of getting any of it back. I was mentally and physically drained. I had given my all for nothing in return and I had nothing left to give. I was so ill myself that I could have done with a hospital bed. He didn't pull with me once. If he had shown a scrap of cooperation I would have stood by him through anything. He was too self-centred for that, though.

Karl came back from his trip to London on December 22nd. That night I went to bed as usual and he stayed on the sofa bed downstairs. In the early hours of the morning, I came downstairs to use to toilet, and almost fainted at the sight that awaited me. Despite my desperate attempts to help him and his unfailing agreement to cooperate, Karl had had a binge to end all binges. It was like a slap in the face. The walls were smeared with disgorged chocolate and cake. It looked like a dirty protest in the Maze prison.

You can imagine how this scene affected me. There were biscuit wrappers, cake wrappers, and chocolate wrappers everywhere. The furniture was so badly smeared with this gunge, that it was hard to tell its original colour. There was half-regurgitated slop that had been spat out, and had landed on the floor, all over the bed and on the bed linen. It's hard to explain the chaos. I didn't even know he had any money for a binge. I demanded to know where he got the money. He was very reluctant to tell me at first. Eventually he told me that he got it off Ray. He said that he told Ray that I wanted a big Christmas present.

I was astounded at this. Nothing could have been further from the truth. I never wanted anything from Karl except his cooperation. To tell his friend that I had more or less demanded a present was the last straw. I'm afraid to say that that's when I lost it. Feeling the way I did, having gone through so much, having had so many heart to hearts with him, having given him so much of my money, my love and my time, something inside me just snapped. I was so mentally and physically ill that I couldn't take anymore. I screamed like a fishwife. I told him that I just could not take any more. I grabbed him and kept shaking him and asking him why he did it. Why did he have to ruin my life? I'd lost my family, my job, most of my money, everything. I'd had enough of his lies and his deceits. I'd had enough of the things he said behind my back. I couldn't trust him. I told him to get out.

He kept saying, 'I've got nowhere to go, I've got nowhere to go.'

I said, 'I don't care. I can't take it any more. Just get out. Get out of my life once and for all.'

He was pleading with me, crying, and begging me not to throw him out. It was too late. I was in such a temper that it was lucky I didn't strangle him. Instead, I kept screaming at him. 'GET OUT, GET OUT, GET OUT.'

When he realised that his begging and crying were not getting through to me, he started banging his head against the wall. Eventually he split his head open. His head was pouring with blood, so that now there was blood on the walls mixed in with the cake and chocolate. I was in a state of panic. Karl was covered in blood, he was also heavily drugged or drunk or both, and my flat looked like a horror film set. I phoned for an ambulance. I felt so alone and so desperate, that I also phoned home. That was probably the worst thing I could have done, but I was not responsible for my actions by then.

It was six o'clock in the morning. Julie got out of bed to answer the phone. I wasn't making much sense, and I was screaming almost incoherently that Karl had split his head open and an ambulance was coming and that I couldn't take it any more. Julie said that she and Dad would be on their way. Well, for Dad to get out of bed at six in the morning would be a first. He must have rushed however, as he and Julie turned up at the same time as the ambulance. I think that was the first time that Dad had set eyes on Karl. If looks could kill!

Dad and Julie stayed at my flat to secure it, while I went in the ambulance with Karl. All through the journey, Karl kept pleading with me, 'Don't leave me. Don't leave me. It will all be different. I'll try harder.'

I said, 'I've heard it all before. We've been together for six years and you never try. You'll never change. I'm not going to take it any more.'

The ambulance pulled up at accident and emergency, and they took Karl in to get his head stitched. As soon as Karl's head was treated, they took him onto St. Julian's ward, which is the psychiatric ward of St. Albans City Hospital. Karl begged me not to section him. The staff told me that if Karl had nowhere to go and no one to look after him, they would be able to section him and keep him on St. Julian's ward. However, if I agreed to take him back, then they wouldn't keep him in.

Dad arrived on St. Julian's ward as this choice was given to me. Dad was all for Karl being sectioned and he gave me an ultimatum. He said that I could go home and they would look after me for Christmas, but only if I washed my hands completely of Karl. It broke my heart to have to leave Karl on a hospital ward for Christmas, but I needed help myself. Even the most selfless person reaches the end of the road. I had certainly reached the end of the road. It was a dead end. Nevertheless, to this day, I am still ashamed and upset at what I did that Christmas. I signed the form saying that Karl would have to stay in St. Julian's ward over Christmas.

Karl was begging, crying, and clinging on to my leg. It was horrendous, but I was strong enough to just walk away and leave him there. I went home to Mum and Dad, supposedly to be looked after. Of course, it wasn't the panacea that I hoped it was going to be. There were so many problems at home, my dad being the root cause of most of them; plus the fact that I was upset and distressed at abandoning Karl, meant I couldn't be at peace or happy. It wasn't long before I started regretting my actions and thinking that maybe I'd done the wrong thing. I went to bed that evening and slept for about 24 hours, such was the measure of my exhaustion.

During that time, Karl constantly phoned pleading to speak to me, only to have Mum or Dad slam the phone down on him. He eventually got me the next evening, which was Christmas Eve. There were carols playing on the TV, peace and good will to all men, and there was Karl, locked on a hospital ward at Christmas because of me. I was in tears. He told me that he had no underpants, no shaving gear, no money, nothing. I couldn't just sit there, but how could I go to the hospital with his things without feeling the wrath of my dad.

Julie was going to Mass on Christmas day, so I pretended to Mum and Dad that I was going with her. Instead, she took me round to my flat where I picked up his things, then took me on to the hospital. She dropped me off there, and then went on to church. She would pick me up after the service. I felt bad deceiving Mum and Dad, especially on Christmas day, but what else could I do. I couldn't see him with no one and nothing. He had just lost his father and his mother said that she couldn't cope with him any more. He had no one apart from me. I still have guilty pangs about what I did, even after all these years. However, I was very sick and under an enormous amount of pressure. I just couldn't take it any more. I loved Karl through it all, but our love could never be. We were both too ill, like two drunks propping each other up.

Julie and I went back to see Karl a few days later. Afterwards, we went to a shopping centre to try to cheer ourselves up. Again, there were carol singers, Christmas lights, and the hustle and bustle of people shopping after Christmas, taking back the singing socks that Aunt Flo bought them, and it just seemed like another world. It was as though I was viewing this scene through plate glass. We were in hell, but surrounded by people having a wonderful time. Ironically, because the scene was so unreal, so bizarre, Julie and I ended up laughing hysterically.

Christmas day had been awful, with Dad having turns and his obsessive compulsion controlling his life. Mum got more and more irritated because she couldn't cope and she was fed up with Dad and with the extra stress that I brought her. The thought kept going through my mind, 'I've had enough. I don't want to go on living.'

I find Christmas time hard, even now. You see the scene on TV, with everyone standing around a log fire, happy and laughing, toasting each other with mulled wine and eating a mince pie, but in my experience, it's not like that. In my experience, Christmas is about stress, expense, and spending weeks walking round shops trying to find presents for people that they don't really want. In return, they buy you a present that you pretend you like, only to have to return it to the shops a few days later. Singing socks are funny for about two minutes. Not only that, but for someone like me who has a food problem, Christmas is like putting an alcoholic in an off licence for a week.

The temptation is just too great. I always look forward to the New Year, with hope of a better life and an end to my problems. I may be fooling myself, but without hope, what have you got?

After a few days at home, I was anxious to get back to my flat. Being back at the family home brought back all the memories of the problems there. I felt as though I was back to square one, after I had fought hard to leave all that behind me. I returned to Martins Court, only to be reminded that my problems followed me everywhere I went. I still couldn't cope alone in the flat. The mess that Karl made was still there. It had set like concrete and so I now had that to deal with. Despite that, despite everything I went through with him, I desperately missed Karl and still loved him.

I used to spend my days doing what limited housework I could cope with in the mornings, before heading off to St. Julian's ward in the afternoons to see Karl. There had to be more to life than this.

THE PETER DALLY CLINIC

I regularly saw Mavis my social worker and I was under a Psychiatrist from Edinburgh House. Whenever I saw either of them, their opinion was the same. I needed a proper relationship. They said that I didn't know what a proper male/female relationship was. They said that I needed someone to cope for me and to look after me. Granted, I had an intense relationship with Karl, and it was true that I loved him, but we were more like soul mates. That wasn't enough. I was in my mid thirties and had never experienced sex. Even my GP, Dr. Gorton, said that if I wanted to get better I should, 'Have a roll in the hay.' It was true. I desperately needed a normal life. If only I could find someone who would look after me and protect me. I thought of Tony.

Tony was a neighbour of mine at Martins Court. He was quite good-looking and a little bit older than I was. He was a lorry driver. I only really knew him to say hello to when we passed each other in the corridors. One day I was walking along the country lane at the back of my flats when I saw Tony coming in the other direction. We stopped and talked and he mentioned that he hadn't seen Karl in a while. I told him that Karl was very ill with anorexia, and that he was currently in hospital. He seemed interested at what I was saying, so I just kept on talking and gave him a potted version of my life with Karl. As we parted, Tony said to me that if I wanted any odd jobs done around my flat then I only had to ask. As it happened, I had some blinds in my flat that had broken and so I asked him if he would fix them for me. He said that he would and we arranged a time. He duly arrived at my flat, fixed the blinds then made a pass at me.

As before, I was flattered that a man fancied me. I was missing a physical relationship, but I was also missing company. I was extremely vulnerable mentally; I had gone through hell with Karl. I thought that perhaps this man might solve all my problems. I couldn't have been more wrong. Why could I never get it right?

I resisted him on that occasion, but Tony was not going to give up. He was a predator and he knew that I would give in eventually. One day he saw me in the car park, and told me that he had just decorated his flat. He asked me if I would like to go round and have a look. The fact that he could decorate made him more attractive to me, as decorating was a big problem in our family. Although I was attracted to him, and he was quite good looking, I eventually realised that all he saw in me was someone that he could have sex with. He was a bully and a brute, (like Chris), and in hindsight I could have ended up in hospital like Karl. I found out about him in the months to come.

Tony had been in the army, The Parachute Regiment, in fact. On his discharge, he worked as a painter and decorator. He was also an alcoholic. He got involved with a girl who thought that there was more to the relationship than there actually was. They were living together and she thought that they were buying a house together, but according to Tony, he was paying the mortgage and she was paying him rent. He said that the only reason her name was on the mortgage was for tax reasons.

One day Tony said to this girl that he was going to America for a couple of weeks to go to a friends wedding, and that she should carry on paying the bills until he got back. Off he went to the States, and his two-week holiday extended to a year. Meanwhile, the girl he left at home was feeling a bit miffed at having to pay all the bills including the mortgage, while Tony swanned around America having a good time. She eventually stopped paying the mortgage and moved out. When Tony came home, he found that he very nearly had his house repossessed. He was so incensed at this that he tracked the girl down at her brother's house. When she opened the door to Tony, he grabbed her and started beating her. Her brother tried to protect her, but Tony laid into him to such an extent, that he crippled him. The man never walked again. Tony was duly arrested, and went to prison for grievous bodily harm. He was a bad lot all round, and I ended up with him intimidating and abusing me for eighteen months. I lost my virginity to this brute, and he took it like a prize. I can't half pick 'em.

Out of loneliness, desperation, and a desire to get a better life, I did many things that I was, and still am, ashamed of, and I'm sure my family were ashamed of me as well. I was certainly disloyal to Karl, whom I still loved despite everything. I can make no excuses, except to say that I was very ill. I wasn't coping and in fact, I was barely surviving. The depression was black and the eating was consequently out of control. Really, I should have been in hospital. When you're in that state, you think that there's no lower that you can sink. You feel that you're at the bottom of the trough, and that the only way to go is up. Yet, however low you sink, there's still lower you can go. I have cried for hours and hours alone, thinking about how low I had sunk.

I was missing Karl desperately, despite the crap I took while he lived with me. That's the extent to which I hated being on my own. I couldn't be on my own. I hated my own company and I hated myself. Therefore, in my mind, it didn't matter what I did for company and what they did to me, it meant that I wasn't alone. It didn't matter because I didn't matter. I was repulsive and worthless and felt lucky if anyone wanted to spend some time with me, regardless of how far down the food chain he was.

On one visit to Karl in hospital, he asked me if I could sell his car for him. Karl owed a lot on credit cards and, like a mug, I paid the interest on them when he was in hospital. Karl was an expert on credit cards. He would use one to pay off the other, then not bother to pay off the first. He would move on and leave his debts behind. When he asked me to sell his car for him so that he could put the money in a building society account, I thought that maybe he was changing for the better. Maybe he did want to try to pull in my direction.

I sold the car to Barbara's son for around £300. As he was allowed off the ward from time to time, Karl came with me to the building society to open the account. I was very excited about his change of heart, and I said that he should pay his benefit into the account as well. I said that if he tried, I would help him any way I could. He hadn't changed. The minute my back was turned, he drew all the money out to spend on his problem. Would I ever learn?

A few days later, I had an appointment to see Dr. Gorton and Karl agreed to accompany me. On our way to the surgery, Karl said that he wasn't going back to St. Julian's. That was all I wanted to hear. I went in to see Dr. Gorton, and he asked me how I was and whether I needed more pills. I broke down in front of him. I told him that Karl was refusing to go back to hospital. I told him that I didn't know what to do, but he was very calm about it. He called Karl in and spoke to us both. Karl was crying and literally on his knees begging me to let him come back to the flat. I couldn't let him back. It was only a week or two since he was at my flat banging his head against the wall because I couldn't cope with him any more. Nothing had changed.

Dr. Gorton told me that I should go and that he would take care of Karl and take him back onto St. Julian's ward. I was trying in my poor way to do what was right and best for Karl. Dr. Gorton recognised that. He said to me that what I had to contend with would be hard for someone without any mental health problems. He could see that life with Karl was just making my condition worse.

I left his office in tears. On the one hand, I wanted Karl back because I was lonely and desperate for his company, but on the other hand, I knew that we'd be back to square one. Dr. Gorton left a waiting room full of patients and drove Karl back to St. Albans City Hospital.

I knew that Karl needed help, and that had to be professional help. I couldn't help myself, let alone him. Although St. Julian's ward wasn't geared to eating disorders, (after all, it was just one ward of a general hospital), it was better than nothing. If nothing else, they may have been able to refer him to a specialist unit.

During this time, I had been in contact with David Britten. He told me that he was trying to pull strings to get Karl into The Peter Dally Clinic, which he ran. However, if Karl were to have any chance of getting in, it would be much easier if he were still on a psychiatric ward, rather than in my flat. Of course, the best laid plans of mice and men often go awry, as they say. Shortly after Dr. Gorton took Karl back to St. Julian's, there was a ward meeting. They decided that as Karl was no longer banging his head against the wall, he was cured and could be discharged. According to their records, that was what Karl had been admitted to hospital for. They were washing their hands of him to free up a bed. Therefore, a few weeks after going into hospital, Karl was back home with me. He had nowhere else to go.

I told Karl that he needed proper help for his problems. He eventually agreed that if I could get him into David Britten's unit, he would go voluntarily. I phoned David to tell him this, but he said that at the moment he was having funding difficulties, and that I should look into other possibilities in the meantime. With that in mind, I looked into a unit that was part of the Royal Free Hospital. Karl and I went to look at the unit, but unfortunately, the waiting list was for months. The woman who ran the unit told us that as the list was so long, people were dying before a place became available.

A few weeks later, David Britten invited Karl and me along to the Peter Dally Clinic for an interview. David obviously knew Karl and knew how Karl forever bucked the system. He looked at Karl and said, 'If I take you onto my unit, will you work with me this time? There are dozens of people who could benefit from being here, and I don't want to waste a space on someone who won't work with me.'

Naturally, Karl agreed. Karl always agreed. He would promise you the Earth, if that was what you wanted to hear.

David took me to one side and said, 'I'll take Karl, but I'm doing it for your sake. He's pulling you down, and you need some space so that you can sort your own problems out. Karl is incurable. He will always be an anorexic, and there is very little I can do for him. On the other hand, there is a chance for you. Away from Karl, you have a chance to have some sort of a normal life, albeit somewhat limited.'

So, Karl was admitted to the Peter Dally clinic in Victoria. Each patient had his or her own room, which made it nicer but it also made it more open to abuse. Karl abused it for all he was worth. Soon after Karl went in, David Britten phoned me. He told me that if Karl was to recover, I should cut all ties with him. He said that was also the only way that I would ever get a semblance of a normal life. He said that if I packed up all Karl's things, he would store them for me.

I knew it made sense, but that didn't make the decision any easier. I finally decided to take David's advice. Karl had quite a few belongings, but I had no way of getting them to the clinic. I phoned Kay in Swindon to ask her advice. Kay seemed to understand my decision and reasons behind it. She told me not to worry about transport, as Karl's uncle had a van and he would come and help me with the big stuff. However, she said that Karl would need some of his personal belongings and clothes at the hospital. I said that I would take them around myself the next day. I thanked Kay for her help, but I begged her not to tell Karl what I was going to do. I said that it would be best all round if it was a clean break. She promised that she wouldn't.

The next afternoon, I went to the clinic with Karl's things. My intention was to leave them at the hospital entrance. When I got there, I saw Karl sitting on the other side of the door. Apparently, he had been there all day. Kay had gone against her word and warned him what I was going to do. Once again, I was greeted with Karl on his hands and knees, crying and imploring me not to leave him. I tried to explain that it was for the best, but he kept on saying that he couldn't survive without me at least visiting him.

I caved in. Once more, Karl's emotional blackmail had triumphed. Mavis, my social worker, once told me that Karl could play me like a musical instrument, and I think she was right. I carried on visiting Karl on a regular basis.

From time to time, I saw David Britten whenever he was free. I liked and admired David. If I'm honest, I also fancied him. He was in a position of authority and he'd helped me a lot. This scenario had many similarities to the one with Les from Hill End. I hoped that it wouldn't end like that. David would phone me at my flat from time to time. I was always very pleased to hear from him. He had a wonderful charisma. He called me Susie, constantly asked how I was and was very charming. He was also flirtatious when he spoke to me, almost as a boyfriend would talk to a girlfriend. I was always boosted by that. Such was my low self-esteem; I was boosted and flattered by any half-decent man who spoke kindly to me. On many occasions, he said that I was an attractive woman and that he was attracted to me. I knew that many of the girls who encountered David were madly in love with him. I think that he knew that and enjoyed the buzz he got from it, although I didn't think there was anything more to it.

One day, David called me into his office. He locked the door and said to me, 'I think you've got something to tell me.'

I went bright red and said, 'I don't know what you mean.'

He said, 'I think you do. I want to know how you feel. If you were to tell me how you felt about me, that wouldn't be a wrong move.'

I cringe at it now, and it was obvious that he was getting off on this. I said, 'Well I do think a lot of you and I am attracted to you, but I don't know what your personal situation is.'

I was very wary after all that I went through with Les. I didn't want the same thing again. David went on, 'Well, ask me anything and I'll answer you.'

I said, 'Well, do you have a wife?'

'No.'

'Do you have a girlfriend or any children?'

'No.'

I said, 'Well, who do you live with then?'

He said, 'I've got a house in Acton that I share with my brother.'

That was true, although I was later to find out that he only lived in the house during the week in order to get to work easily. At weekends, he went home to a place in the country that he shared with another man. Of course, I knew none of that at the time.

Then he asked, 'So, how do you feel about me? You want a future, don't you? You want a life after Karl. Tell me how you feel about me.'

I repeated what I told him, in as much as I found him very good-looking and that I got excited when he phoned me. I went on, 'But you're a very important and attractive man and you can have your pick of women. I don't want to get hurt again.'

He said, 'I promise you, I'll never hurt you.'

I didn't know what to think. I got up to leave and went over to give him a hug. As I did so, he didn't reciprocate, but instead his body stiffened. I should have realised in that instant that he was not attracted to me, and that it was all a mind game.

Nevertheless, as I left he said to me, 'I'll be in touch. You haven't done the wrong thing telling me how you feel. You can ring me at any time, and I'll be there for you.'

I floated home. Here was someone with tremendous charisma, who did an important job, who professed an interest in me. Coincidentally, this was around Valentine's Day, so I went out and bought an elaborate card and sent it to him. Of course, I didn't sign it, but waited for him to contact me. Well, I waited and waited. I thought about him morning, noon and night. It was what got me through the crap in my life. I clung to him like a limpet because I was desperate. I still waited, but to no avail. He never phoned me. Eventually I plucked up courage and I phoned him, or at least I tried. Every time I phoned the clinic, they told me that David wasn't there or that he was busy or some other excuse. However, one day, more by luck than judgement, I managed to get him on the phone. He was very offish with me. He wanted to know what I wanted. I just said that I wanted to talk to him, but he said, 'Don't you know I'm a busy man? I can't keep taking phone calls from you.'

Naturally, I was devastated. I had been suckered once again. He had what he wanted, he had his buzz, but obviously, he had moved on. Having said that, every six months or so, he would ring me. He would say that he wanted to know how I was getting on, but really, it was as if he wanted to keep the fire alight. He wanted to keep my dependency on him. Really, I should have told him to sod off. But of course, I didn't. I was always pleasant on the phone to him, as I was when I saw him while visiting Karl. You can be too nice to people.

In the summer of that year, my sister Julie and I decided to go on a 5-day coach holiday to Yorkshire. We both desperately needed a break. Julie was very sick by now. As her life at home continued, so her OCD exacerbated. She had obsessive religious scruples and she was in torment over the mistakes she thought she had made in her life. Her illness was not, and to this day, is still is not admitted to nor recognised by either herself or any of the family. Mum and Dad already had one mentally ill daughter and they didn't want another one. In fact, it was typical 'burying your head in the sand' syndrome. If it was ignored, it didn't exist. If a doctor was unable to look at Julie, then she wouldn't end up in a mental hospital as I did.

Paradoxically, I was the lucky one. I got help of a sort. Yes, the Maudsley was a hellhole, and admittedly, no medication has cured me to date. However, I have been able to come to terms with my illness, I can openly admit to it, and further more, I am not getting any worse. As with many psychological illnesses, alcoholism for example, the first stage of recovery is actually admitting you have a problem. That's not to say that everyone can be or will be cured, but it's a vital first step.

Julie's religion was not giving her any peace, either. Everything was black and white to her. In her eyes, her sister was 'sinning' with men. She thought that if I carried on the way I was, then I would be sure to spend eternity burning in hell.

Therefore, we went on this coach holiday because we thought that we could help each other and have a break from everything. Karl wasn't too chuffed at my going, but I told him that I needed a break. I promised him that I would ring him a couple of times while we were away, and I gave him a copy of our schedule, just so that he could think of me each day and imagine the places we visited.

I wasn't physically up to the rigors of a coach holiday, as apart from anything else, I was constantly tired. You have to follow an itinerary, which means early starts. I wasn't very good at early starts. I'm still not. I would have been better off in a bed in a nursing home, but I went to try to help Julie as much as anything. Julie did her best to help me, despite her own problems. She went out and bought me some 'Blue John' earrings. Apparently, Blue John is only found in the Castleton area, and is the rarest natural formation in the British Isles. Bless her; she spent the last of her cash on them for me. I still have them to this day, and I treasure them. She was forever buying me coffees to try and perk me up and she was also constantly in health shops, trying to find me a magic potion to try and make me well. She did what she thought was right to help me. However, at the same time, she was also very distressed by the life I was leading. She knew more about me than any other member of my family did, although she didn't know the full story.

One day, we went for a walk round the local area, and Julie found a Catholic Church. She discovered that there was confession taking place that evening, and decided to attend. I don't know what was said as confession is a private thing between you and the priest, but clearly I was discussed, as Julie said that the priest would see me the next night. When you're sick and troubled, and you're in agony of mind, you cling to any straw. If someone told me that standing in manure would help, I would be the first in line at the stable with my shovel. Because of that, I agreed to go along and meet the priest in his presbytery the next evening.

When I got there the priest didn't know who I was or that I had an appointment to see him. He was very offish with me. He said, 'Well what do you want then. What have you come here for?'

I said, 'Well, my sister spoke to you last night in confession and you told her to send me along to see you.'

'Well, I can't remember asking anyone to send you along,' he said, 'I know nothing about you.'

I felt small and humiliated. Because of his attitude towards me, I didn't really go into too much detail of my problems. I didn't feel he would be overly sympathetic towards me. After speaking to him, he just trotted out that I should go to confession, attend church regularly and atone for my sins. Basically, he was saying that if I didn't, then there would be no hope for me, and I would burn in eternal damnation. Not something you want to hear when you're sick and need help.

I walked back to Julie in floods of tears. To make matters worse, when I saw her, she told me that there had been a phone call at the hotel from Karl. She said that he was in a distressed state, and that he would ring back later. That was all I needed. He must have gone to a lot of trouble finding out our hotel phone number, because even we didn't know what it was, baring in mind that we moved every day on this touring holiday. Holiday? That's a laugh.

Anyway, he duly phoned back that evening. The essence of the phone call was that David Britten was going to throw him out of the Peter Dally clinic the next day. He said that he didn't know why. He said that David had just come up to him and said that there was no hope for him; there was nothing more that they could do. He was crying on the phone, saying that he had nowhere to go and didn't know what to do. I tried to tell him there was nothing I could do. I said that I was on this holiday with Julie and that I was unable to get back, and even if I could, there was no way that I was going to leave Julie on her own.

Expert manipulator that he was, Karl then changed tack. He told me that he'd made an attempt on his life by taking an overdose, and he had been taken to accident and emergency where he had his stomach pumped. The inference of that was that if I didn't take him back, he would do it properly next time. I knew that Karl was a liar and a conman, but he was counting on the fact that I was a soft touch, and he knew what strings to pull. He knew that there was no way that I could prove or disprove what he was saying. However, I was strong. I stuck to my guns and told him that I couldn't get back before the end of the week, and that he would have to try to help himself this time.

As for Karl's 'unwarranted' expulsion, I later found out from David Britten that Karl had been abusing drink while he was on the unit, and that he had warned Karl on numerous occasions that it wouldn't be tolerated. Karl ignored the warnings and went on in his own sweet way, doing whatever he wanted. One night, he came onto the unit drunk. David did a spot check on his room to find alcohol stashed away, as well as chocolate and cakes. David told me that he was so angry that night that he didn't want to make a snap decision. However, he said that he had no choice but to expel Karl the next day, as it wasn't fair to the people on the waiting list for his clinic. He said that Karl had just thrown everything away, and thrown everything that he tried to do for him back in his face.

Needless to say, the rest of our holiday wasn't a bundle of laughs. I was worried about Karl, naturally, as that's my nature. Julie thought that Karl shouldn't have phoned and put extra pressure on me. She said that once again, he had abused the help given to him and was expecting me to bale him out. Julie was anti Karl anyway, and said that he was self-centred and only thought about himself. That's undoubtedly true, but that is the nature of the illness. I can identify with that. People with Karl's problems have little or no chance of overcoming them.

Overall, the holiday was a waste of time. Julie and I were of no real help to each other. Julie did the best she could, but her nagging at me to change my life and pray over a religious artefact couldn't help my problems, and at the same time, her problems couldn't be helped by me, owing to the fact that she didn't admit to having any. She still says that there is nothing wrong with her, and that she only has to 'pull herself together.' If only it were that easy.

When we got back from our holiday, we found that Karl had been given a room above what can only be described as a brothel. Opposite the flat was the seediest, spit and sawdust pub you could imagine. I used to visit him once a week and I was horrified at the scenes I saw. People constantly rolled out of the pub and threw up on the pavement, then staggered over the road to the flat below Karl's, to take advantage of the 'facilities' there. The music from the flat below was so loud that it used to shake the windows. It was disgusting and dingy, and full of fleas. Karl was regularly bitten. I felt so sorry for him, that he had come to this. I blamed myself, as is my nature. I also used to beat myself up, as I should have been able to clean the place up for him, to make it fit for a human being to live in, but of course, I couldn't. Nevertheless, I did what I could for him.

I visited weekly, and took him provisions and bought him phone cards, so that he could keep in touch with me. I no longer gave him money, as I knew that he would abuse it. Happily, the seedy room was only a temporary stopgap, and Karl was eventually allocated a flat in Shepherds Bush. He didn't want to move there, as he wanted to come back with me. He still thought that I would take him back. That could never be, however. I told him that we would always be friends and that I would stand by him. I promised him that I would never desert him. However, I told him that we could never live together again. With my problems, I found it hard enough coping with life. When I had Karl's problems added to that, life became impossible. I didn't like leaving him on his own. For all his faults and failings and the trouble and heartbreak that he brought me, I still loved him. That may be hard to understand for an outsider, but that's how it was. We may not have had a physical love, but we certainly had a strong emotional love, at least I know that I did.

On the other hand I needed someone 'well', to look after me. I needed looking after as much as Karl did and I didn't want to spend the rest of my life on my own. I told him that I was going to do something about it. I was going to join a dating agency.

THE DATING GAME

I would be lying if I said I wasn't nervous about joining a dating agency, but I was determined to try to see if I could find an answer to some of my problems. The question was which agency I should join. There are hundreds. In my cockeyed way, I tried to do the right thing and went for what I considered as 'safe'.

I found out that the Catholic newspaper, The Universe, ran a dating agency. I suppose I was naïve, but in my innocence I thought that if I joined one run by a Catholic organisation, I might meet someone who had certain principles and standards. I told Mum and Julie what I was going to do. They weren't over the Moon about it, but they agreed with me that if I was going to join a dating agency, then better if it were a Catholic one. I didn't tell Dad. I didn't dare.

I wanted someone who would accept me for what I was, and not use me or treat me like crap. Yet another wrong move. As Del boy would say, 'What a 22 carat plonker you really are.'

All of the men that I contacted or who had contacted me had a 'check list' of what they were looking for. They wanted a woman in full time work (and on a good income) who owned her own property and who had no health problems. I was none of those. Therefore, I didn't meet any of those men.

Not to be downhearted, I kept looking in the Universe, and one day I saw a promising advert. It was from a man of around my age, who said he was loyal and sincere, and was looking for companionship from a similar type of person. There was no mention of wanting someone who could run ICI, or someone who was training to be an astronaut, so I thought that I might be in the running. I plucked up courage and wrote to this man, and we arranged a meeting.

Our rendezvous was in Westminster Cathedral, in Victoria. Quite an innocuous meeting place, I thought, so I felt quite confident. When I saw the man, I wondered if he had just come down from the bell tower and I was the replacement for Esmeralda. All right, I'm being very unkind here. He wasn't that bad, but he was as short as he was round, (only coming up to my shoulder), with a moggy eye and breath that could peel paint. I thought, well you're no oil painting yourself girl, and you've got all your problems and illnesses, give the poor man a chance. We decided to go to the local Army and Navy café for a cup of coffee. He said that he was so excited as he had never had coffee in a department store before.

As we sat and drank our coffee and he proceeded to tell me his story. He said that he was lucky to be able to meet me at all. He told me that he had to get up at 5am in order that he could meet me at 2pm as he normally he spent Saturdays washing and colouring his mother's hair, doing the shopping and doing the housework. He went on to say that if we got married, we would have to live with his mum. He said that although he hadn't told his mother about me yet, he was sure that if he broke the news gently, and that I joined the Catholic women's guild, and joined the same prayer group as her and jumped through other hoops, in time and with the wind in the right direction, he was sure that she would come to accept me, and as long as I spent my life taking care of her every whim she would allow me to live under her roof.

I know, I know. I should have run a mile, but being Susan Kennedy I felt for the underdog once again. I thought, what a crap life you're living. It's as bad as mine. From what I could gather, his mother was an embittered woman who ruled his life with a rod of iron. He did everything around the house, and jumped to her every command. He said that he was a junior clerk in an insurance office, and that in ten years he would get either a small pay rise or promotion to deputy tea boy. So we had that to look forward to. He said that we would have some time to ourselves if we did get together, as his mother went to the Catholic prayer group every Wednesday night, so we would have two hours alone then. Yippee!

He said that he didn't mind that I didn't have a full time job because I would spend all my time at home being a constant companion to his mother.

I was staring at this man, trying to imagine him with a personality. He certainly didn't have a sense of humour, because none of this was funny. I should have just jumped out of the window and ran like the wind. Instead, when he asked me if he could see me again, I said yes. He was on cloud nine. He said that he had never travelled as far as St. Albans.

He came to my flat, and we prayed together in the front room, although I suspect that I was praying for different things than he was. Afterwards I walked him back to the station. It's an awful thing to say, but he was such a bore and his breath was so bad, that even though I was desperate and needed someone to look after me, I really couldn't take that on.

The thought of meeting his mother sent shivers down my spine, so I took the coward's way out and wrote him a letter saying that we couldn't really make a go of it. He wrote back and said that he was heartbroken at this, and that he had to go to Lourdes to get over me. In view of the fact that we had only met twice, it made me realise how many sad and lonely people there are out there, and what terrible lives they lead.

Although it has been levelled at me since that I should have persevered and found a 'good Catholic man', none of those men wanted a 'reject', (apart from 'moggy eye').The only thing that we would have had in common was the faith, and I was only clinging onto that by my fingernails. Besides, going to church doesn't make you a Christian any more than going to a garage makes you a mechanic. For that reason, I decided to give up on the Catholic dating agency. I joined an agency called 'Perfect Match'.

Two men who belonged to MENSA, the high IQ society, started this agency. I don't know if I was fooling myself, joining this agency. After all, I consider myself a prime candidate for DENSA. Nevertheless, join it I did, in the hope that I would find someone who was slightly less shallow than my previous encounters.

With Perfect Match, you're sent a list of people with their profiles, and you pick who you would like to meet. Well, from the first list I received, I saw a man whom I thought sounded nice. I phoned him up and we agreed to meet by the bottle bank. I know, start as you mean to go on. Anyway, he turned up in his car, and when he got out, the first thing that came into my mind was Charlie Drake. He was the image of him, right down to his curly blond hair. The only difference was that this man was as Irish as a peat bog with an accent to match.

As a complete novice in this dating game, I stood in full view of the car park, so he saw me as he drove in. Anyone else would have hidden behind the bottle bank to see what the man looked like, giving themselves an option to leggit. Mind you, I'm not like that. I would never hurt anyone's feelings. I know from painful experience what it is like to be rejected. I should have been more honest with them, and told them at the end of the date how I felt. My dad always said that I should grow a shell on my back.

This man came over to me and introduced himself. He said that he didn't know where to go, so I suggested The Galleria, which is a shopping complex in Hatfield. I can see now how naïve I was, getting in a car with a complete stranger, but I always try to see good in people. I think God must have been looking after me, on more than one occasion.

We arrived at the Galleria, and he said, 'Well, what do we do now?'

I said, 'Well, we could go for a pizza, if you like.'

He then said, 'I haven't been out for a meal before. You'll have to show me what to do.'

Although I was quite used to showing my special needs students from Oakland's things normal adults take for granted, I expected a little more from someone who was a potential husband. After arriving at the restaurant, (and showing him how to wait to have a table allocated to us), we eventually sat down. I could see how excited he was at being here with me. He was practically bouncing up and down in his seat. The waiter then brought the menus, and he looked at it as if it was the operating instructions for a nuclear reactor. He said, 'What do we do now, then?'

I said, 'Well, you read the menu and decide what you would like to eat.'

He said, 'The thing is, I'm not really used to eating out. I get most of my meals by the roadside hot dog caravan.'

I said, 'Well, I'm going to have a serve yourself salad, from the salad bar.'

He said, 'I've never been to a serve yourself bar before. What do you do at a serve yourself bar?'

'Serve yourself,' I replied.

I took him up to the serve yourself bar, and explained in minute detail what you did. Anyway, we got our meals and returned to the table. He then explained to me that he had a wife at one time, and lots of money and a big house. He said that he had his own business as a builder and labourer, but that his wife had left him and taken everything, and that he now lived in a caravan in a field. He said it was a nice caravan and it had a pipe connected to the cold water supply outside. I thought for a minute that he was going to say that he had a pipe connected to his car's exhaust.

He went on to say that he had employed a secretary, and had given her some money to go out and buy a word processor, but that that was the last time he had seen her. It sounds funny, but at the time, I felt sorry for him. He had obviously had a rough life.

He said that, as he was on his own, he never had any incentive to spend any money, which was why he was living in a caravan. However, he said that if I stayed with him, he would give me anything that money could buy. Of course, he never had any money, but I wasn't going to be cruel enough to tell him that.

After the meal, we returned to his car. Sitting in the car, he turned to me and said, 'What's it to be then. Are you going to go out with me again?'

To be honest, I was too frightened at that stage to say no, because I was a long way from home. If I had said no, he may have turned nasty or just refused to give me a lift back, so I said yes. A great big beaming smile lit up his face, and I could see that he was on top of the world. I know I shouldn't have said that I would see him again, but I didn't want to hurt him. Besides, he had paid for the meal. Such was my lack of self worth in those days; I believed that if someone paid for something for me, I owed him or her something. You have to be cruel to be kind, isn't that what they say? I sometimes wish I could be.

He drove me home to Martins Court, and he said that he was looking forward to seeing me again. He was so enthusiastic and said that he could build his life up again and that he wasn't feeling depressed anymore. I said goodbye to him feeling awful. He drove off with that Charlie Drake smile, and I felt like a heel. I knew that I wouldn't see him again, and I should have had the courage to tell him.

A couple of days later, I was walking back from college and he pulled up beside me in his car. The smile hadn't left his face, and he went on again about how I would transform his life and that I could help him with his business. He asked me if I wanted a lift home, but I declined and made up some excuse that I was visiting someone. He drove away, but I was quite frightened. He obviously knew where I worked. What would he do if I told him that I didn't want to see him again? I had seen enough violence with Chris and Tony, (who was still pestering me at this time, by the way).

I decided to ask Julie for her advice. She, naturally, was horrified at my story. In her view the fact that he wasn't 'a good Catholic man', was bad enough. She said that I should end it now, before things got out of hand. I asked her if she would help me, and phone the man on my behalf, and she agreed.

A day or two later, I was walking home from college, and there he was again in his car. I was very frightened now, as I didn't know what to expect. He wound his window down and said, 'I was very hurt and upset that you've done this to me. You led me on. You led me to believe that we had a future together. Now all I've got is the caravan.' He went on, 'You're turning down someone who would have idolised you and loved you and given you everything.'

Of course, I was in a terrible state after that. I didn't mean to hurt him. I know that I should have told him after the meal that we were not a match. I went home in floods of tears. I was worried that he would come back and pester me, but to his credit, he didn't and I never saw him again.

Apart from Perfect Match, I also used to read the dating ads page from the local paper. This took the form of a chat line. The idea is that you read the person's profile, and then if you liked what you saw, you phoned them. Again, I know I was putting myself at risk in answering these ads, as you have no way of knowing if the people were who they said they were. In reality, these were not so much chat lines as sex lines, composed by people who only wanted uncomplicated sex and one night stands. Then again, people who join dating agencies are not wired up to a lie detector when they fill the form in, otherwise most of them would never get any further. I know that there are many genuine people who join dating agencies. The trick is to wheedle them out from the predators.

One of the men that I thought was genuine was a police officer from Devon. I phoned him up and he sounded nice and told me a bit about himself. He said that he was the only police officer in the village where he worked, and his job was mainly to man the phones. He said that he had a panda car, and if someone had their bike nicked, he would race to the scene and deal with it.

However, if there was a major crime, like a window had been smashed or someone had not paid their TV licence, then he had to phone the next village to get the assistance of the bobby there. Very 'Heartbeat'. Consequently, he had a lot of time on his hands and access to a phone, and so had plenty of time to phone chat lines. I later found out that firemen did the same thing. I wonder if their wives knew.

Over the course of several conversations, he told me that he had left his wife for the woman who lived opposite. It seems that the woman, (who was married), had a nice house with a built in sunken Jacuzzi. The policeman, by all accounts, would go over from time to time, to try out said Jacuzzi and anything else that came to hand. He said that his own marriage had gone stale, and this neighbour of his opened up a whole new world for him. A world of rampant sex, by all accounts. He had to be careful in carrying on this affair, because obviously she only lived opposite. So he used to pretend to go to work, and then nip round the rear entrance of the woman's house, after she had left a sign in the window that her husband had left for work.

After a while doing this, he decided that he wanted to make the arrangement permanent, so he left his wife. However, the woman was not so keen to leave her husband, saying that he was a good provider and she didn't want to hurt him. The upshot was that the policeman ended up in a bed-sit, hence the chat lines. He said, quite honestly, that he wanted a woman like his neighbour who would give him the same excitement that she had given him.

I know what you're thinking. I should have told him there and then that I was not exactly what he was looking for and left it at that. But you see, he sounded nice on the phone, and my two and a half brain cells weren't working up to speed. I did tell him that I was somewhat limited, and tried to explain why, and he said, 'That's all right. If you're the right one for me, I'll help you overcome any problems.' If only he knew.

We decided to send each other a photo. I received his photo and he looked quite an attractive man, with dark hair and a beard, and very smartly dressed. I liked what I saw, and I thought in my naïveté that he might like the look of me. Despite my often negative opinion of myself, I had to admit that I wasn't bad looking.

The next day, I was walking round the shops, looking at all the couples buying plants for their gardens and bits and pieces for their houses, and I thought, that's what I want. I don't want to be roaming round on my own. I want to be part of a normal relationship. I was on a high as I walked around, as I thought in my innocence, that maybe the policeman and I could have a future together and all my problems would be solved.

I got home to see my answer phone flashing. It was from him, and the message said that he had seen my photograph, and he was sorry but I wasn't the one for him. Obviously, I hadn't ticked all of his boxes. Once again, I had been rejected. Immediately all my suppressed views of myself came to the fore again, in other words: ugly, repulsive, unlovable and a thousand other adjectives. Looking back, I realise that he had a picture in his mind of what an ideal partner would look like. It is a very shallow template on which to base a relationship, and I'm sure that in time he would realise that. Maybe women who didn't like beards, for example, would reject him. This may sound nasty, but I hoped that someone would reject him, just so he knew how it felt. I was an expert. I had been rejected all my life.

Ever a fighter, I phoned another man. He was a widower, and he said that he was a writer and a songwriter, but because he hadn't sold anything, he worked in a corner shop. He used the shop phone to ring the chat lines when he had no customers. Over time, he told me all about his tempestuous marriage. He said that he had two children with his Malayan wife, who had been a staff nurse in a psychiatric hospital. He said that his wife was very unstable and was prone to fits of temper. (A psychiatric nurse who was unstable? Never heard of such a thing.)

He went on to say that they were forever having violent rows, during which she would physically attack him. In fact, he became a battered husband. He said that during one of her rages, she had cut off one of his testicles. Now, he never let on to me why he had allowed that to happen, or indeed how one of his testicles had became available to be cut off during a row. Nevertheless, there it was, or at least, there it wasn't!

He told me that these rows became more and more violent, (though goodness knows how), until one day, his wife killed herself. He said that he was now trying to rebuild his life, while at the same time caring for his children. I agreed to meet him, (you knew I would, didn't you?) but we didn't have very much in common and so nothing came of it.

As you may have gathered, I wasn't having very much luck in this dating game. I knew my friend Dana had joined one a few years earlier, so I asked her to share her experiences with me. What she told me didn't exactly fill me with confidence. Dana said that one man she went out with didn't have a car, so she offered to give him a lift to their date. Again, not something that you would recommend in this day and age. Anyway, the man got in the car and Dana drove off. As they were travelling along, she noticed that the man didn't have his seat belt on. She suggested that he put his belt on, just to be on the safe side. Well, this man did no more than to wrap the seat belt around his neck. He then tried to fit the buckle into the clasp, nearly decapitating himself into the bargain. Dana was terrified that if she had to brake fast, the man would strangle himself. She spent the rest of the journey looking out of the corner of her eye at this man who didn't know how to put a seat belt on, thinking, 'Oh God. I've got to spend the rest of the evening with him.'

They managed to get to their destination without the man hanging himself. She said that somehow she got through the evening, but despite the fact that she wanted to just drive off with smoke coming from the tyres, she asked the man if he wanted a lift anywhere.

He said, 'Yes please, could you take me to my house?' which she agreed to do, hoping that it wasn't very far. As they pulled up outside this man's house, she noticed the curtains pulled back and there was an elderly couple peering out.

He said, 'Oh, that's my mum and dad. Would you like to come in, because they want to meet you? They'll have the cocoa on.'

Much as the invitation was almost too good to turn down, Dana made the excuse that she had to go, as she had to get up early in the morning. She said goodbye to him and left half a pound of rubber on the road as she drove off.

On another date, she actually met the man in the car park of the pub, so at least she didn't have to give him a lift or be a party to death by stupidness. Dana bought the drinks and they sat down. After a while, he said that he was going to the toilet. So Dana sat there sipping her drink waiting for him to come back. Well, 10 minutes went by and no sight of her date. 15 minutes turned into 20, and still no sign. Dana thought that he must have had some sort of stomach upset and hoped it wasn't catching. After half an hour, she decided that she had to find out what had happened to him. She went to the toilet entrance and asked a man who was going in, to see if her date was all right. The man came out and said that there was no one in there.

Deciding to call it a day, Dana went into the car park to get her car. It so happened that her car was parked outside the rear of the toilets. As she got in her car, she looked up and noticed that the gents' toilet window was wide open. It didn't take Hercule Poirot to work out that far from having the runs, the man had got cold feet, climbed out of the toilet window and just run. Suffice to say, there wasn't a follow up date.

I suppose everyone who has been a member of a dating agency has a horror story to tell. Nevertheless, I couldn't let that put me off. I desperately wanted someone special in my life. Daily life for me was one long round of illness, non-coping and stress. I was still constantly harassed and bullied by Tony. A strong man with me would have put a stop to that, if nothing else.

I frequently visited Karl at his flat in Shepherds Bush. We never discussed my ventures in the dating game. He didn't really approve, but he never tried to put me off. The truth is, I still loved Karl, and it was the highlight of the week when I visited him. However, we could never be a couple. He was too ill for that. His illness was all encompassing and he only had time for that. I would always come in second place.

Things were not too good on the work front, either. I had been missing days and arriving late on the occasions I did turn up, so in fairness to Barbara and the rest of the staff, I asked for a sabbatical. Barbara suggested that I had a word with the head of the personnel department, which I did. The personnel manager was very nice to me and said that she understood what I was going through as she had gone through bad times herself. She finished by assuring me that my job was safe, and that she had received good reports about my work in the department and they didn't want to lose me. She said that I could come back whenever I felt able to.

I felt very reassured by that meeting. It never crossed my mind to get anything in writing as I trusted Barbara and I felt that I could trust the personnel department, after what the manager had just told me. How wrong could I be? When I eventually went back about six months later, they told me I had no job. The head of personnel had gone and been replaced by someone whom I had never met. She knew of no arrangement that had been made between her predecessor and me. All my work colleagues, the tutors and especially Barbara, acted as if they never knew me. I had no support from any of them. Apparently, there had been big changes at the college, with redundancies and people fighting for their own jobs, and it seemed as if speaking up for me would have put their own careers at risk.

I went to a staff meeting which turned out very embarrassing. No one stood up for me, even though when I worked there they all said what a good job I did. Even Barbara, whom I considered a friend, said nothing at all and just sat looking at the floor. That hurt the most, as I had done a lot for her, including going through a horrific court case. I ended up breaking down in front of them when I tried to defend myself. That always happens when I try to stand up for myself; the tears come. I knew how good I was with the students, and so did they.

I walked out in silence, and that was end of my time at Oakland's. I was very happy there, and I knew that I had made a difference to the students. I never praise myself up; in fact, I'm forever running myself down. However, I do know that I was good at my job, and so did Barbara and her staff. It hurt me that the seven years of good service that I gave meant nothing to them.

Back to the dating and I went out with one or two others. One was quite a young boy who was a football fanatic. He spent the entire evening talking about football. He went to great lengths trying to explain the offside rule to me. I didn't have the heart to tell him that I didn't know the difference between the offside rule, the off stage rule or the off-the-peg rule.

If that was bad enough, another man I met had a fascinating interest in bricks. He could tell you anything you ever wanted to know about bricks, and that evening he did. He even had a collection of bricks at home. For all I know he even named them. I was tempted to say that I had a collection of my own and that they were holding my flat up, but I didn't.

One of the last men I met was a dumper truck driver. He was quite good looking. He said that he had been engaged to a girl, and that they were buying a house together. One evening he looked out of his bedroom window to find her 'engaged' with his best friend, so that relationship broke up. Obviously, he was trying to find a replacement for his fiancé. Although we went out two or three times, he wasn't right for me.

I was quite disheartened about this dating business now. I was sitting in the kitchen at the family home talking to Mum about it. I told her of the men that I had met and the disappointment that I had experienced. Mum wasn't too surprised at that. I think that she was of the opinion that if the man didn't come from a good Catholic home, then he wouldn't be right for me. I didn't agree with her though. I have seen too many bad Catholic marriages, where the couples stick together just because of the faith. I knew that there had to be more to a relationship than that.

Mum told me to give up on the dating agencies and to trust to fate. I said that there was one more contact from Perfect Match. I said that I had received a letter from a man who sounded nice, and that I would like to meet him.

'All right then,' said Mum, 'just one more then call it a day.'

'OK,' I said.

'What's this man's name, anyway?' asked Mum.

'He's called Dave,' I said.

DAVE

The letter that I received from Dave was unusual in many respects. It was the only letter I received from a dating agency, for one thing. In all the other cases, either the men had phoned me or I had phoned them. Very few people went to the lengths of writing a letter. The other thing that came across to me was the sincerity in the writing. It was a genuine and very open letter. I thought that if the person writing this was as sensible, level headed and sincere as his letter, then I just had to meet him.

On the evening of 14th May 1997, I phoned Dave, who was a lorry driver living in Aylesbury. A down to earth cockney man answered the phone. Right from the start, we seemed to be speaking the same language. Far from coming across as suave, sophisticated, and indeed pretentious, as many people are on the phone, it was refreshing to talk to someone so relaxed and informal. He was very easy to talk to, and we spoke for a long time on various subjects.

One of the things we had in common was our hatred of the Christmas parties that we both suffered as children. Together with the fact that we both hated having to call complete strangers Auntie, (even the men!) and not liking the pantomimes and holidays on ice. It seemed that we had known each other for years, instead of 5 minutes.

I told Dave that I was due to go out with the dumper truck driver that evening. I said that it depended on how that date went on whether I saw

Dave or not. I had already more or less decided that I didn't have much in common with dumper truck man, and that we wouldn't be seeing each other again. However, in fairness to him, we had already arranged to meet and I didn't want to let him down.

I did meet dumper truck man that night, but it wasn't very successful. Again, I took the cowards way out and left a message on his answer machine saying that I wouldn't be seeing him again. The next evening, the phone rang and it was Dave. Dave had a similar accent to dumper truck man, so that's who I thought it was. I was a bit embarrassed as I thought that I would have to break the news to him that I didn't want to see him again.

I said, 'Oh, hello. Didn't you get my message?'

'No, what message?' he asked.

I said, 'Well, we had had a nice time together during our dates, but I don't think there is a future for us.'

Back came the reply, 'But we haven't had any dates. You only phoned me for the first time last night.'

That was when I realised my mistake, and knew that it was Dave. I thought that he must be keen, as he had sent me a letter and now followed it up with a phone call. He told me that he was off the next day, (Friday), and asked if we could meet then. I decided that it was better to grab the bull by the horns and go for it. The longer I left it, the more nervous I would become. I agreed to meet him the next day at my flat, and gave him directions. I know I shouldn't have. I can imagine there are women reading this with their toes curling up, thinking how stupid it was to invite a complete stranger round to my flat.

The next day, Dave phoned me on his mobile to say that he was five minutes away. I watched out of the corridor window to see his car arrive. As he got out of the car, I could see that he was carrying a large bunch of flowers. This was unknown in any of the other dates I had been on. In some cases, I even had to buy the drinks in the pub. I was so touched by this kind thought that I gave him a kiss on the cheek. I led him up to my flat and showed him to the living room while I made him a cup of tea. As I put the kettle on, I turned round to see Dave propped up in the doorframe, chatting to me. He seemed so relaxed and laid back, that it actually put me at my ease. I made the tea and carried it into the living room, and we both sat down. I felt very comfortable and calm with this man sitting there. So relaxed, in fact, that I started telling him a potted version of my life story.

I thought that it was best if I told him about myself, so that he knew what he was letting himself in for. I didn't want to get fond of him and then go through the humiliation of rejection further down the line. I have always believed that honesty in a relationship has to come first.

Well, that conversation went on for hours. I told him everything; all about my limitations, my problems, Karl, I left nothing out. In fact, I wish I had written this book back then; it would have saved me a lot of time. I even told Dave that I had a commitment with Karl, and that I would stand by him whatever happened and I would never let him down or reject him as a friend. Much to my surprise, far from running out of the flat screaming, Dave took all this on with quiet composure. He wasn't at all fazed by what I told him.

After all the ear bashing I had given Dave, I suggested that we went for a drive to Shaw's Corner, the former home of George Bernard Shaw, which is in Ayot St. Lawrence. One of the negative traits that I found with Dave was that he seemed a bit abrasive. This was something that I would have to get used to, as obviously he would have to get used to a lot about me. For example, on our way to Shaw's Corner, I tried to direct him. He said, 'I know where Shaw's Corner is. I drive round here all the time.' I thought then that he was quite sharp.

Then, when we arrived at Shaw's Corner, and I mentioned what a nice area it was, he merely said, 'Oh, it's alright. But I've got just as good a view where my house is.'

There's for and against to this. It was obvious that he had no 'bedside manner'. I wasn't going to get flowery language and 'shall I compare thee to a summer's day', but on the positive side, what you saw was what you got. He would tell it like it was, and he was not going to be a con man. He wasn't going to tell me one thing, but then do the opposite behind my back. I had a lot of that with Karl, who would talk softly and say what you wanted to hear, but the minute your back was turned, do the reverse. The difference in characters would take a lot of getting used to. I have since come to realise that much of Dave's sharpness stems from nervousness. Far from being cool and collected all the time, he was quite shy. That shyness manifested itself in an abrasive manner.

One part of his personality that I loved was his sense of humour. As we walked around Shaw's Corner, he had me in stitches regaling a story of how his family went to Glasgow for his niece's wedding. He drove everyone up there in a minibus, and everyone was allocated a couch or floor to sleep on. Dave got a room that was in the process of being built, so he slept on a couple of bags of cement. Suffice to say that he didn't get any sleep, despite the fact that he had been up since the early hours.

Came the time of the wedding, he drove everyone to the church, and then on to the reception, which was held in the basement of a pub. There were no windows in this place, but when he asked why they were having it there, the answer was that the best man knew the owner, and so they got it cheap.

Half way through the evening, Dave decided to check on the minibus. A big Scotsman stopped him on the stairs and asked him where he was going. Dave told him, and this Scotsman said, 'No, it's alright. You can look later. Go back to the party.' Dave insisted on going, so the Scotsman reluctantly stepped out of the way and Dave carried on up the stairs. When he got to the minibus, he was shocked to see that it had been broken open and all the possessions had been taken. Some money was stolen, a couple of credit cards and a few items of clothing. He ran back to the party and noticed that the aforementioned

Scotsman was no longer there. Dave told everyone what had happened, so all the guests went up to search for the criminals. You can imagine the sight, a dozen wedding guests in their best attire, roaming the streets of Glasgow looking for the thieves. Anyway, they couldn't find them, so went back to the pub to phone the police.

Everyone was fed up now and said that they all wanted to go home. That of course meant Dave had to drive them. Baring in mind that he had been up for 36 hours, they still wanted him to drive them all home, which would take at least 8 or 9 hours.

Anyway, he got them all home safely, which was the main thing. The next day Dave was watching the wedding video, which he shot. He said that he filmed the speeches and then just set the camera on a tripod and let it run for the rest of the evening, until the film run out. As he was watching the video, he noticed the best man doing sign language to a guest behind the camera. Ten minutes later, he did it again, and then breathed a sigh of relief. Just then, there was a shot of Dave, obviously on his way to check the minibus. It was obvious that the best man was in on the robbery, and from the sigh of relief, he knew that it had all gone to plan. Dave gave a copy of the video to the police who interviewed the man, (who had a record, by all accounts), but they said that there wasn't enough evidence to charge him, although they were sure that he was part of it.

The way he told the story, in a deadpan way, was hilarious. Fancy going to a wedding and being mugged by the best man. Anyway, realising that this man had a sense of humour was a good sign, as I too have a good sense of humour. You have to, being me.

After our walk, I thought that Dave would drop me off at my flat, and that would be the end of our date. However, he had other plans. He said that he would like to take me out for a meal. He had already told me that he was doing this lorry driving work, and that he had been there years and was reluctant to move on, even though the wages were quite poor. Therefore, I knew that he wasn't flush with money, and so I didn't want him spending what little he had on me. Nonetheless, he insisted, and so I told him of a nice pub restaurant in the area called The Wicked Lady. As we drove into the car park, he asked my advice on where we should park. I helpfully directed him to a nice quiet spot at the far end of the car park, well out of the way of any other cars or indeed lights. You see, I had been used to Dad who could only park in the space normally reserved for a jumbo jet. It hadn't sunk in yet that Dave was a professional driver and could park his Granada in a shoebox.

After our meal, we walked back to the shady nook to get the car, to find that the boot had been forced open and the spare wheel had been stolen, along with all the tools. I stood there anticipating the blow-up that would have inevitably happened with my dad. It didn't come. That was another major plus about Dave's personality. Dave said later that it cost him £100 to replace the spare wheel. He never asked my advice about where to park after that.

We returned to the car park of Martins Court, Dave switched off the engine and looked nervously at me. 'What do you think,' he said, 'would you like to see me again?'

A beaming smile lit up my face and I said, 'Yes please.'

He matched my smile, and said that he felt like he'd known me all his life. I then asked him in for a cup of coffee. Dave didn't know me well enough then to know that when I said coffee, I meant coffee. He thought I meant naughtiness, so he declined. I appreciated him for that, as so many others had tried and often succeeded in taking advantage of me. We kissed goodnight, and so ended our first date. It had lasted nine hours. I floated back to my flat that night. Perhaps this was the one after all.

The next day, things seemed very different. I recalled the conversation that I had with Dave in his car the night before. I told him that I was thinking about moving from my flat, so that I could get away from Tony. Dave told me not to worry about looking for another place, as I could move in with him. He also said that I was the girl that he was going to marry. Things were moving too fast for me. I couldn't think about moving away from St. Albans, where my family was, where all my friends were, plus my GP and social worker. I certainly couldn't think about marriage. Although we had spent nine hours together, mostly speaking about my problems, I was sure that Dave couldn't know what he would be letting himself in for with me. I came with a lot of baggage. What if I gave up my flat to move in with him, only for him to reject me when he realised what he had got? What would I do then? It was true that I liked Dave. Nevertheless, I wasn't prepared to be hurt again, and I thought that Dave didn't deserve to be hurt by building his hopes up. He deserved better than me.

I wrote him a 'Dear John' that day, explaining everything and that although I liked him, I thought that we didn't have a future as I was too sick. I was unable to make any commitments for a future with neither him nor anyone else. I posted it thinking that would be the end of it. There would be no more dating agencies. I couldn't put anyone else through that, and I didn't want to go through it, either.

Dave was having none of it. He wrote back saying that he fully understood what I was saying, but that he deserved a chance to prove that he wasn't like all the others. He said that although he was sure that I was the right one for him, he knew that I had to take my time in coming to the same conclusion. He went on to say that if we stopped seeing each other now, we would never know if we were right for each other. He said that we both deserved a chance to find out. I agreed, and phoned him to arrange our next meeting.

We went out on a few more dates, but then a couple of weeks later I got cold feet again and sent him another 'Dear John'. I felt that he was getting too keen. I told him that I was limited in what I could do, but he said that it didn't matter. He could cope for me. He said that if I were to move in with him in Aylesbury, I would have a much happier life.

Although it was true that I was unhappy alone in my flat, I was unable to make the move. Part of my illness was that my mind changed from one day to the next, or even from hour to hour. Part of me wanted to go in an instant. However, an inner voice kept telling me that it would be the wrong move. All my life, I went along with what everyone else wanted. I wanted to make everyone happy. I would agree with people, then instantly regret it. If I was to leave my 'safe' life in St. Albans, I had to be 100% sure that it was with the right person. At that moment, I was not sure.

During the early part of our courting, Dave got several 'Dear John' letters and phone calls attempting to end things. To give him credit where credit's due, he was still sure that I was the right one for him. He must have seen something in me that I could not.

Meanwhile, Mavis my social worker had organised for a girl to come round to my flat in Martins Court, to supervise me doing housework, as part of cognitive therapy. The girl had very little idea about what to do, and she had even less idea about my problems. She used to come to my flat where I made her a cup of coffee, and she sat there saying, 'Well, what do you want to do then?' I would then try to run a vacuum round or do a bit of dusting, while she sat and watched. It didn't really work. I used to get more worked up over the fact that she was coming to my flat, than I did when I had to do it on my own. My nerves were in a terrible state before I even got round to tackling the housework. To give credit where credit's due, at least Mavis was trying to help me.

When Mavis and the rest of the team heard about Dave, they were naturally worried, given my previous history with other men. Their idea was that I should be in a protected environment, where I could learn to cope on my own, and get a bit of a backbone. So that instead of reaching out to men as a lifeline, for protection and a solution to my problems, I would eventually go into any relationship as an equal. They realised that I had many problems to overcome before I reached that stage.

With a view to that, and also because I had so much trouble living in my flat, Mavis took me to a group home, for people who were psychiatrically ill. We arrived at this group home around teatime, and the first thing that struck me was how dirty and unkempt it was. There was not much in the way of staff in this place, because the housemates were deemed able to cope to a large degree, by themselves. However, they needed the protection of a communal set up that was overseen by staff.

We walked in to find fag ends everywhere, the carpets dirty, the chairs all soiled. There was a man in the kitchen cooking the dinner, with a cigarette in his mouth with six inches of ash hanging off the end, threatening to drop into whatever concoction was in the pan. As I looked round the kitchen, I could see that the cutlery and plates lent themselves to the rest of the decor, which is to say they were none too clean. I thought to myself that although I have a phobia with cleaning, nevertheless, I still have very high standards. I like things to be neat, clean and tidy, and despite all my problems, my flat was neat, clean and tidy.

I couldn't bear to live in grime, mess and chaos, which I would if I came to live in this home. Apart from that, most of the people that I could see in the home seemed to be in a far worse state than I was. They were very drugged, and most seemed to spend a large part of their time staring at a television screen. Some mumbled away to themselves, while some didn't talk at all. In addition, their personal hygiene matched their surroundings.

I cried when I came out of the house, because I thought, It's come to this. They're deciding to put me in a home like this. There was a bit of me that thought that, despite my many problems, I was worth more than that. I just knew that there was a 'normal' person inside of me, wanting to come out. I knew that I wasn't mad, but that I had problems coping, and I needed to be understood. I needed someone to find a way of helping me cope. I knew that I wouldn't find it in a home like that. I told Mavis that I didn't want to go in, as I didn't think that it was suitable for me. Of course, officials of any kind get quite angry if you don't take up their suggestions. I couldn't help that. I still had some say in how and where I lived. They would just have to keep me on their books a while longer.

Mavis then suggested a place called Artisan Crescent. This was a small block of housing association flats, supervised by MIND, the national association for mental health. The measure for getting one of the flats was that you had to have a psychiatric illness, although at the same time, be capable of living on your own. All tenants would be given one hour a week support and counselling from a MIND community worker. On the practical side, an officer from the housing association visited every two weeks to deal with leaking taps and so forth, and to give advice on paying bills.

I went for an interview for a place in Artisan, but I was not successful. I was disappointed, as it sounded like a good compromise to me. I would still have my independence, my own front door key, and pay my own rent, but on the other hand, I would be free from Tony and I would get the support that I needed.

However, as luck would have it, within a short space of time, another vacancy cropped up. Again, I went for an interview, and this time I was accepted. I went along to look at the flat with Alison, who was the MIND community worker assigned to that block. I liked the flat straight away. It was a block of six flats, and mine was to be on the ground floor. It was smaller than Martins Court, but much brighter. I asked Alison why the flat had become vacant.

'Has nobody told you?' she asked

'No.' I said

'Well, the girl who occupied this flat committed suicide in the bedroom. Would that make a difference to you accepting the flat?'

'No, it's alright', I said, 'I'll take it.'

The flat was to be completely redecorated for me, and the previous tenant had put in new carpets just before she died, bless her. The flat didn't do her much good. I hoped that wasn't a bad omen for me.

Both Mavis and Alison were keen that I didn't tell anyone that I was moving, apart from my family. They wanted me to have a fresh start away from all my previous troubles, and to learn to live by myself. That included Dave. I did tell Dave, however, although he wondered why I would want to bother moving to a new flat at all, when I could move in with him. I stuck to my guns though, because I wanted to try to make it alone, and I thought this was the best bet. I also thought that Dave still didn't realise the full extent of my problems. I thought that if I burnt my bridges and moved in with him, and then it didn't work out, that would leave me with nothing.

Mum and Dad agreed with my decision. They thought that if I moved in with Dave, it would just be a bolthole. They also thought that Dave was too persistent, and that he should have given me more space. They didn't really want anything to do with him. It was nothing personal; they were just looking out for me. I don't think it would have been fair on Dave, either. I was very unstable at the time, thinking one thing one minute and another thing the next. The number of 'Dear Johns' that I sent him were testament to that.

Dave was very good about the whole thing. In fact, he moved me into the flat, with help from Dad and Julie. He even put the curtains up for me and built some shelving in my cupboards. Julie said that it was very good of Dave to help me, him being 'just a stranger.' Far from being a stranger, Dave was becoming more and more integral to my life. All I needed now was to overcome my myriad of problems. Perhaps the new flat would help.

David Hooper

ARTISAN CRESCENT

After I moved in to Artisan Crescent, it didn't take very long to get to meet my new neighbours. It was a very close community and I soon found out that everyone looked out for everyone else. We were all as vulnerable as each other.

A girl called Jackie lived upstairs. She had a boyfriend called John who lived in Hemel Hempstead, and would stay with her two or three days a week. John was an alcoholic, and he'd met Jackie in a psychiatric hospital where she was being treated for Bipolar disorder, otherwise known as manic-depressive illness. John was in there trying to come off the drink. John always maintained that there was nothing wrong with him and he took every opportunity to tell Dave, 'There's nothing wrong with us two, it's all the others.' He used to distance himself from all the others with mental health problems, because as far as he was concerned, alcoholism isn't a mental health problem.

Moving on a bit, after a couple of years, Jackie decided to move into John's flat in Hemel. Whilst the relationship worked when John was only visiting Jackie a few days a week, when they were together permanently the situation became intolerable. John's drinking became unendurable for Jackie, they started to argue and the relationship began to break down. As a result, her mental health problems got worse because of the stress. She ended up back in a psychiatric ward suffering from a bad flare up of Bipolar disorder. Meanwhile John drank himself into stupors, and eventually a relative found him dead in his flat.

Jackie then spent a long time in hospital, before eventually getting another flat, near to the hospital.

During the time that I lived in Artisan though, Jackie was doing quite well, as she had a part time job as a dinner lady at a school and did volunteer work in a charity shop, while studying for a degree in German at night. I think that Jackie's story goes to show that it is important to have the right relationship if one has mental health, or any other, problems. The wrong relationship can pull you down, as happened between Karl and me. That was certainly the view of Mavis and Alison, and the rest of the mental health team. The right relationship can make all the difference, whereas the wrong one can be a disaster. The jury was still out on whether Dave was the right person for me.

Another neighbour of mine was a man called Colin, who suffered from depression. He would leave the flat every day looking like a businessman going off for a day's wheeling and dealing. What he actually did was to go to the library to write copious letters of complaint to various authorities. That's all he ever did, complain. I think they based Victor Meldrew on him. He was always miserable, which is understandable if you have black depression, but he would also have mood changes. For example, sometimes he would let Alison and the housing officer into his flat, and sometimes he wouldn't. Now, it was part of the deal of us having these flats, that once a fortnight a housing officer would visit, and once a week you got an hour's counselling from a MIND caseworker. I didn't have very much to do with Colin. Whenever he met anyone, he would try to solicit him or her to complain about whatever his hobbyhorse was at the time, which was mostly about mental health problems. I'm not the complaining type; I just like a quiet life.

Another neighbour was a man called David. David suffered from schizophrenia. The story was that David had developed the illness by taking illicit drugs in his teenage years. He had elderly parents who visited him practically ever day. His dad had Alzheimer's, and so just sat in a chair. Meanwhile his mum would clean his flat and prepare his meals. When they went home, they took his washing and brought it back ironed. To outsiders, for example Alison and Mavis, it looked like David was doing very well, because they were never around when his parents were there doing everything for him. Whenever I saw Mavis, she would tell me that one day, if I was lucky, I would be as efficient and independent as David was. However, David did far less than I did and was less independent than I was.

Another neighbour of mine was a woman called Clare, whom I became friends with and we are still friends to this day. Clare was a seventh day Adventist and had married a seventh day Adventist minister. Soon after their marriage, they immigrated to America, and very shortly had two children. Clare told me that she was always a shy, retiring type. She said that although she tried hard to fulfil the role of the minister's wife, and all that it entailed, it was extremely difficult for her and she felt that she didn't do it particularly well. Her husband made it abundantly clear that she didn't do it very well.

They travelled around from state to state, trying to live up to her husband's ambition of attaining dizzy heights in the ministry. He never moved up in the hierarchy, and subsequently blamed Clare for it. He said that if he'd had a more dynamic wife, it would have made a difference to his promotion prospects.

Sometime during her thirties, Clare started to get ill with the onset of schizophrenia. She became less able to cope with everyday household chores, not to mention the ministerial wifely duties. Her husband showed no Christian compassion or care during this time, but instead would berate her about what she hadn't done.

As time went on, Clare started hearing voices, losing touch with reality and all the other symptoms associated with schizophrenia. Her husband told her that he was going to leave her for a year, in order that she sorted herself out. He said that if she hadn't pulled herself together by that time, then the marriage would be over. That left Clare on her own, suffering from a severe mental problem, trying to bring up two children. Eventually, Clare's children had to be taken away from her, as she couldn't cope.

The husband came back after a year. He had spent that year having an affair with one of his parishioners. When he saw that Clare was even worse than before, he left her and promptly sold the family home. Not only did he leave her, but he left the children as well, leaving Clare to foot any bills that came in for them. Obviously, she couldn't work, and so had very little money coming in. She had to live on the money from the divorce settlement, and so ended up in a seedy little rented flat, hardly seeing her children at all.

She realised that her only course of action was to return home to England, where at least she had access to a benefit system. She moved in with her elderly parents. This was not ideal, as her parents were quite old and in bad health themselves, and were unable to cope with a sick daughter. Her parents decided to move to the coast and not long after, her mother died. Clare then spent some time in a psychiatric hospital, before getting the chance to move into Artisan Crescent.

The last of my neighbours, and certainly by no means least, was a man called Mark. Mark had been bullied all his life, starting when he went to nursery school at the age of three. He was a sensitive, feeling, gentle person, and of course, the bullies realised this and capitalised on the situation.

A very intelligent man, he got top A levels in pure maths and applied maths. He went on to college to do a HND in engineering. It was at college when he had a massive breakdown, and could not continue with his course. There were many similarities with me. His illness manifested itself in paranoia, an inability to cope, avoidant personality disorder and depression. He spent a long time in and out of hospitals, before moving into a group home. He then shared a flat in Martins Court before being offered one of the places at Artisan.

Mark became one of my fondest friends, and we still keep in touch to this day. Mark is a gentle and genuine man who has been blighted with a terrible illness, and I'm proud to call him my friend.

Dave and I were still seeing a lot of each other, spending weekends together, either in Artisan or in the Pastures, his house in Aylesbury. We decided to go on holiday together to Cornwall, as he knew it quite well. He didn't have much money, and in fact, the most we did on our weekends together was to go out walking. However, he said that he could afford a weeks self-catering in Cornwall if I would like to come, and I agreed.

I had mixed feelings about going. I wasn't sure that I could hold together for a week, and in fact, Mavis my social worker was certain that I wouldn't. Nevertheless, we went to Newquay and it was lovely. The same couldn't be said about the accommodation, however. The place was supposed to have been highly rated by the tourist board. We think that the owner showed the inspectors his own house, and not the garage in which we stayed. Yes, it was a double garage converted into a flatlet. What made it worse, this garage was at the bottom of such a steep incline, that you almost had to abseil down to it. Coming out in the morning needed stamina, ropes and a team of Sherpas!

Because it was at the bottom of this hill, naturally that's where all the water ran. The place was damp, dank and smelly. The bed linen smelt like someone had been ill all over it, so we used our coats as blankets. The place was filthy and badly needed decorating, or failing that, demolishing. The shower was disgusting, with mould and mildew growing out of every orifice. The water that dripped out of it was as cold as ice, not that we wanted to use it. I wondered if Dave had used the same holiday brochure as Dad. I wanted to cry, but even more, I wanted to go home. How was I going to cope here? I hated mess and dirt, but I was unable to clean up.

Dave came to the rescue. He made the place habitable for us, and cleaned everywhere. He carried me through that holiday, in order for us to have a nice time. The actual holiday was nice, it was a lovely area, the weather was good, and Dave showed me some beautiful spots. It was just unfortunate that we had to end up in that dive every night.

The day we were due to go home, Dave had a surprise for me. He said that he was upset about the rotten accommodation we had, and that he wanted to make it up to me. He said that he was going to take me to a four star hotel for a night, just so that I could experience a bit of luxury, before going home. He couldn't really afford it, but he insisted.

We went to a place called the Hotel California. This was more like it. Lovely bedrooms with en suite, a top class restaurant, indoor swimming pool, gym, table tennis, bowling alley, and all extremely clean and inviting. We were both looking forward to a nice, romantic evening together. It didn't happen. After our four-course meal, which was lovely, we wandered off to the lounge to soak up the atmosphere. There was an announcement that there was going to be a quiz, and anyone could take part who wanted to. I didn't really want to take part, as I had no confidence in things like that. I was still on antidepressants and other medication, and so my brain was not as sharp as it once was. However, Dave said he would like to take part, so that's what we did.

We did the quiz, and while the papers were taken away to be marked, I turned to Dave and said that I wanted to phone Karl.

'What for?' he asked

'Well, I told Karl that I would be home tonight,' I explained, 'and so he'll be waiting for my phone call. Don't forget, he's all alone in that flat and he'll be counting down the hours and minutes to hear from me.'

Dave couldn't understand any of this. As far as he was concerned, we were on holiday together, so why couldn't I forget about Karl for one night and enjoy the last night together. I told Dave that I had to phone, because I knew what it was like to be all alone. A phone call can make all the difference. Dave reluctantly agreed, but told me to be quick, as the quiz results would be announced soon.

I went off to make my call, and in the meantime, it was announced that Dave and I had won the quiz. Dave was annoyed that I wasn't there when it was all announced. He is shy and gets nervous when left alone at public functions and that comes out as sharpness and bullishness. It was hard for me to adjust to this abrasiveness. I missed the gentility and suaveness of Karl on those occasions. If truth be told, I wanted to hear Karl's voice as much as he wanted to hear mine.

When I got back to Dave, he could see that I was upset. 'What's happened?' he asked.

'I've just phoned Karl,' I said, 'and he told me that he had taken an overdose and had to be taken to hospital to have his stomach pumped.'

Dave was livid at this. 'He can tell you anything he likes, and you believe him,' he said.

'Why shouldn't I believe him?' I asked.

Dave replied, 'Because he's told you all that before, and you said that you didn't believe it. He can play you like an instrument. He hates the idea of us being together, and he's just winding you up. All I wanted was for you to forget about Karl for one night, and enjoy the rest of our holiday. It's cost enough.'

'I'm going to bed,' I retorted and stormed off. I was livid. He couldn't tell me not to speak to Karl. Didn't he realise that I loved him. If he made me choose between himself and Karl, there would be no contest. It would be Karl every time.

Dave and I didn't speak to each other for the rest of the time we were on holiday, so it wasn't exactly an unmitigated success. He dropped me back at my flat the next day and went home. The holiday was over and I was back to reality. Back to the illness and the problems and the not coping. I didn't know what to do. I do know that I wasn't happy.

A couple of weeks later, I phoned Dave who was at his mum's house. He went and met up with his sisters, Irene and Sheila. Mary, his mum, answered the phone and put me on to Dave. I was in a desperate state, the depression was black and I wasn't coping at all. I asked him to come and get me. He told me not to worry and that he would come straight away. As I put the phone down, I started to panic. Dave was on his way to take me back to his place. Although I couldn't cope in Artisan, I also couldn't cope in the Pastures.

Whenever I stayed at Dave's house, I got terribly depressed while he was at work and I was left on my own. I knew that it wasn't the answer. I didn't know Aylesbury and, apart from Mary and Irene, certainly didn't know anyone in the area. However, although Mary was nice to me, she didn't have a clue about all my problems and illnesses, and I didn't feel comfortable in trying to explain.

I phoned home and told them what was happening. I spoke to Julie and told her that I wasn't well, and that I'd phoned Dave, he was on his way to get me, and that I was panicking about it. About half an hour later, Dad and Julie arrived at my flat. My family felt that my going off with Dave wasn't going to solve anything. They knew that I wasn't happy on my own, but for the same reason, they knew that I wasn't happy at the Pastures. Dad didn't really understand my problems, despite having a myriad himself. He was wild with anger, because as far as he was concerned, I was just causing him a load of worry and trouble, and messing everybody about. Dad couldn't cope with his own life, so the last thing he wanted was crises phone calls from me. He thought I should just knuckle down, and be happy living on my own in a beautifully decorated, newly carpeted, flat.

What he, and everybody else didn't seem to realise, was that I was desperately ill. I was unable to make decisions or commitments. My mind swayed one way then the other. I didn't know what I wanted. Julie felt that Dave was pushing me too hard, and that he should just back off and realise that I was mentally ill, and that there was no way that I could form a normal relationship.

Soon after, Dave arrived into this explosive atmosphere. Dad turned on him straight away, and told him not to keep pressuring me.

'I'm not pressuring her,' said Dave, 'Sue phoned me up and asked me to come and get her.'

'Don't you know she's sick?' asked Dad. 'Why can't you leave her alone?'

'I'm not going to leave her alone. She loves me,' said Dave.

Dad came back with, 'If a gorilla said it loved you, would you believe it?'

Charming! Dad was now comparing me to a gorilla. Surely I had something else going for me than that.

Dad kept asking for Alison's phone number. He thought that she would come and tell me to pull myself together and get rid of Dave. He eventually found her number, but there was no answer. I was glad. I didn't want anyone else involved. Dad had met Alison once. She told him that pills were not the answer to my illness.

'Well what will cure her?' asked Dad

'There's no cure, but the right relationship would help.' She answered.

Was this the right relationship? I didn't know. I knew that I wasn't happy. I was happier when I was with Dave, but if it was the right relationship, then surely I would be happy all the time and would jump at the chance to move in with him. I didn't know what I wanted, and that's the truth. I wanted to be well, and I wanted to be 'normal'. I wanted to be able to cope alone. I certainly didn't want to be surrounded on both sides by warring factions.

Just then, the phone rang and it was Mary, Dave's mum. Dad answered the phone and Mary asked what was going on. Dad said, 'Don't you understand, Susan's ill. Dave's putting her under pressure.'

Mary said, 'But Sue's very fond of Dave and they get on well together.'

Dad replied, 'Don't you understand, she's not in any position to make a commitment, or to move in with anyone. She's psychiatrically ill, and she'll be psychiatrically ill for the rest of her life.' He went on, 'She has to be on her own, whether she thinks she does or she doesn't. She reaches out to people in desperation, but she can't cope with a normal life. She has to be on her own.'

Dave's sister Sheila then came on the phone, and started talking about us loving each other. I didn't love Dave. I was fond of him, but I didn't love him. Sometimes I thought I did, and told him so, as I didn't want to hurt his feelings. However, the love of my life was Karl. Mary then came back on the phone and asked to speak to me. She said, 'What's the matter with you? You're messing Dave around. You're going to have to make a decision and make up your mind what you want.'

I was sobbing by then. I didn't know what I wanted. I certainly didn't want all this. I didn't want everyone getting at me. Didn't they know I was ill? I don't blame Mary or Sheila. They were only looking out for Dave, and from their perspective, it looked like I was messing him around. I wasn't doing it on purpose, I was ill. Everyone was treating me as if I was normal.

'JUST LEAVE HER ALONE,' shouted Dad.

'I'll leave her alone if she wants me to leave her alone,' said Dave, 'but until then it's between Sue and me.'

With that, Dad turned on Dave as if he wanted to punch him. Dave just stood his ground and said, 'I'm not going to hit you Pat. You're 77 and an old man. I'm six foot and a fit, strong young man.'

Seeing that he wasn't intimidating Dave, Dad then turned on me and tried to strangle me. Dave then stepped in and had to physically pull Dad off me. In the ensuing struggle, Dad ended up on the floor by the cooker. Dave then pointed his finger at Dad and said, 'If you ever try anything like that again, I'll put you in hospital.' With that, Julie turned and said, 'Right, I'm calling the police.'

A short while later, a policeman turned up. He asked what was going on, and Julie said that Dave had attacked Dad, but of course, Dave vehemently denied that and told him what had actually happened. I also told the policeman what had happened, that Dad had gone for me and that Dave had pulled him off. Dad kept repeating that Dave was pressuring me to go away with him. He said to the copper, 'Don't you understand? She's mental. This is a MIND home. Don't you understand, MIND, MIND, MIND.' As he said this, he was banging himself against his head. The policeman looked at Dad and said politely, 'Yes sir. I know what MIND is. My son's just done a parachute jump in aid of their charity.'

He then turned to Dave and started talking to him about the follies of parachute jumping, and what a good job MIND did. I could tell that he was on Dave's side. He then asked Dave for his side of the story. Dave told him about getting the desperate phone call from me, and that he had come over as soon as he could. Meanwhile, Dad kept interrupting and saying that Dave was pressuring Sue to marry him and to move away, while Dave tried to defend himself and say that it wasn't like that. The policeman told Dad in no uncertain terms to keep quiet, as he'd had his turn and now it was Dave's.

After hearing both sides, the policeman said that he would like to talk to me alone. We went in the communal lounge and he said to me, 'It's up to you love. Who do you want to go home with tonight, Dave or your dad?'

Well, there was no way that I could go home with Dad that night. He was incandescent with rage and I knew that the row when we got home would be phenomenal. Therefore I decided that I would be safer going home with Dave. At least for that night I knew that I was safe from any more altercations. I told the officer my decision, and he said, 'Well, I think you've made the right choice there love.' We went back into my flat and told everyone my decision. The look on Dad's face broke my heart. I understood that underneath the rage and anger, he was only trying to look out for me, albeit in a cack-handed way. I felt that by choosing Dave that night, I was choosing against my family. Dad just said, 'That's ok, you've made your decision. Take care.' Then he and Julie left, and I drove off with Dave.

I spent the night with Dave, but he had to go to work the next day, leaving me on my own. He had told his mum that I was there, and so the next day she came round. I could have well done without it. Mary didn't really have a clue about my mental health problems. I felt that I couldn't really tell her about myself. I put on a brave face while she was there, but I felt terribly unhappy. As soon as she went, I packed my bags and went home to Artisan. I knew that it was a mistake to go to Dave's in the first place. I knew that I couldn't use it as a bolthole. Wherever I went, whatever I did, I was in torment, because the hell was inside my head. I was ill and needed the support of the health team at St. Albans, plus the support of my family. I couldn't abandon all that.

CHRISTMAS WITH DAVE AND KARL

My relationship with Dave was very unsettled, one minute it was on, the next off. I was fond of him and I liked being with him, but I was still not sure that he was the right one for me. My mind swung one way, then the other, like a leaf blowing in the wind. To be honest, at that stage, if Karl had been well I would have chosen him over Dave as he was the love of my life. Dave was kind, capable and well but Karl and I had several years of history together and had shared an intense emotional relationship.

I still visited Karl on a regular basis, but not as often as I used to, as a lot of my time was spent with Dave; when the relationship was on, that is. However, every time I saw Karl at his flat, I had terrible pangs of conscience. His flat was becoming more and more unkempt and dirty, and it was obvious that he wasn't coping. I felt that I was letting him down, as I was unable to clean up the place and support him as I would have liked but I had so many problems of my own that there was nothing left in my barrel to dredge out.

It got near to Christmas and I found out that he was going to spend it on his own. I had thought that he would have gone to Swindon to stay with his mum, but she decided to spend it at her sister's place. I suspect that she was having a hard time without Tom, and didn't have the strength to put up with Karl's problems over the period.

Mum and Dad had invited me to their house for Christmas Day. They had also invited Dave, but I told them that our relationship was on hold at the moment, but that I would love to go. Mum was very happy about that. She was getting her daughter back for Christmas without the embarrassment of Dave turning up and without Karl ruining things. However, about a week later, Dave and I got back together again. I told him about Mum's invitation, but that I told her we were no longer an item. I said that he would still be welcome though. I had my fingers crossed behind my back when I said it.

I told Dave that it would be better coming from him that we were back together again, and to ask Mum if it would be all right if he still came for Christmas. Dave felt very uncomfortable at doing this. He knew that he wasn't exactly flavour of the month in the Kennedy household, after the ruckus at Artisan a couple of months earlier. Mum didn't believe my account of the row, which was the true account, but instead went along with Dad and Julie's version that it was all Dave. According to them, Dave turned up unannounced, started the row, attacked Dad and took me off to his house, against everyone's better judgement.

Anyway, Dave plucked up courage and phoned my mum. He said that he would like to go there for Christmas, if it was still all right. Well, what could Mum say? She wanted me to go, but couldn't refuse Dave, in case I stayed away and went to his house instead. Dave said that she agreed, but he could hear in her voice that she wasn't happy. I can only imagine the blow up when she told Dad.

With Christmas Day sorted out, I then voiced my concerns over Karl being left alone over the festive period. I knew that Dave would want to see his family over Christmas, and in fact, his sister Sheila and brother-in-law Lajos, had invited him to spend Boxing Day with them at their house in Maidenhead, along with Mary and Irene. I asked Dave if it would be all right if we had Karl over to stay at his house for the rest of the week. Dave said that that would be ok. Sheila found out our plans, and asked Dave if he thought that it was good idea to have his 'rival' round for Christmas. Dave told Sheila, 'I know what I'm doing. If I refuse to have Karl over for Christmas, then Sue will just go to his flat anyway. I would much rather he came to my place, then at least Sue will be with me.' He went on, 'I want Karl to see us as a normal couple. I want him to see that we're an item and that we're serious. He'll give up before I do. I'm going to fight him at his own game, and it's a game I'm not prepared to lose.'

Christmas Day came, and Dave and I went to Mum and Dad's. The atmosphere was decidedly frosty to begin with. To give credit to Dad, he did apologise to Dave about the altercation at Artisan, and Dave shook hands with him and told him to forget it. The situation thawed after that, and we had a nice time.

The next day we picked up Mary and Irene, and drove to Maidenhead to Sheila and Lajos' house. I was very nervous about going, as I didn't know them that well. I also felt that to a certain extent I was playing a part. Dave had believed in being very honest from the outset to everyone about my health problems, because that's the type of person he is. He thought that my family's philosophy of keeping everything hidden was not a good idea. I personally think that somewhere in between the two is the best policy. I told Sheila a bit about my illness, as I thought she would understand, as she has had a few problems herself, and so have her daughters. I don't know if she really understood though. I thought that they might regard me as the mad woman that keeps splitting up from their brother/son. However, the day went quite well, and we all had a nice time.

On December 27th, we went to Shepherds Bush to pick Karl up at his flat. I felt that I was piggy in the middle. I had Dave on one side who, although he never said anything, I could tell didn't want Karl at his house. Then I had Karl on the other side, who didn't want Dave around me at all. They both wanted me exclusively. Karl was not blind, nor was he stupid. From his point of view, he knew it was the beginning of the end. He watched Dave and I go up to bed together each night, and in spite of my doubts about a long term relationship with Dave, he could see that we were serious about each other, and that we were trying to make it work. He knew that we would never be together again except as friends. On a couple of occasions when I was alone with him during that week, we talked about my relationship with Dave. He asked me if I was happy, but in all honesty, I knew that I wasn't. I knew that the unhappiness came from within me. It was part of my illness. You can be sunning yourself on a beach in Barbados and not be happy.

I told him that I still had reservations, and that one minute it was on and the next it was off. I said to Karl, 'Dave's good to me and he's kind and he's 'well', and all of that I need. But he's not as gentle and sensitive as you. I miss that quality in him that I found in you.'

I cried as I talked to Karl. I said, 'I don't really know what I want. I don't want to mess this man around. He's a good, decent, nice man, but I wish I hadn't got involved with him, because everybody's expecting me to act normally, and I'm not normal.'

Karl said, 'Well, you know that I'm always here for you. If you ever want to get away and stay at my flat, you would be more than welcome.' I remember thinking, that's not the answer either. You're in the same state as I'm in, if not worse.

Karl kept his binge eating under control, while he stayed at Dave's. He did have mini binges when Dave and I went to bed, but he didn't mess the place up. If only he could have been like that at my flat.

On New Year's Eve, we dropped Karl back off at his flat. I looked up at the awful grey tower block, and felt terrible. We were leaving him in the mess and filth of his flat, and back to his problems. Obviously, Dave hadn't had the history that I had with Karl, and therefore he felt relieved that it was all over and he could have New Year alone with me. However, for me it was quite different. It broke my heart, having to leave him there. I knew that he would end New Year having a massive binge and probably end it drinking heavily. I thought that, although it was a New Year, there would be no new start for him. He would start the New Year as he ended the last one, with mental problems, living in squalor and in debt. I started sobbing in Dave's car as we drove home. I don't think Dave really understood what the matter was. Didn't we give Karl a good holiday? That wasn't the point. I knew better than most what Karl was going through, and I felt a traitor leaving him. I knew there was no choice, but that didn't help.

Meanwhile Julie, and the rest of my family, had an awful lot of doubts about my being with Dave. They felt that there was no way that I could sustain a normal relationship, and to some extent, they were right. My mind was constantly changing and my moods were constantly altering. To give Dave some credit, he stood by me throughout, where most other men wouldn't. Despite all the hassle, problems and being messed around, he hung in there. He must have seen something in me that I couldn't see. I couldn't understand why anyone would want to be with me.

Dave said to me, that if I stuck by him, he would get me well. He would get me off all drugs and I could live a normal life. If only.

Speaking of Julie, she wasn't at all well herself. She had been asked to leave her job at the benefit office, as she couldn't cope with the work. She then decided to embark on a secretarial course at Oakland's College. She was unable to complete this course, due to her illness, and decided to enrol on a similar course at Pitman's, as it was deemed a less intense course, and one that Julie could cope with. Of course, as with me, the illness follows you wherever you go. Merely going to another place isn't going to alleviate your problems. They come from within, which is where they have to be tackled. The problems followed Julie, and she was unable to cope with the Pitman's course. Eight times out of ten, she didn't even go.

She was also using drink to help get her through the course, and to help with the terrible agonies of mind that she was going through. She also had religious mania, and had bags full of religious relics and holy pictures. Far from her religion helping her, it actually made matters worse. I recognised that Julie was using the only two things she knew to help her through the day. She clung to her religion to try to get her through, and drank to try to ease the pain in her mind. Of course, neither worked. Mum and Dad seemed oblivious to all of this. Julie would wind Dad up by being switched off, when he wanted her to do something, or else she'd be running up and down in her bedroom, listening to music, or talking and laughing to herself.

Mum and Dad were either unaware, or more likely, made themselves unaware that there was anything wrong with her. They lived in denial, and Julie merely said that there was nothing wrong with her; she just needed to pull herself together.

The social workers were all for my splitting with Dave, and told me to cut all ties with him and to change my phone number. They too, felt that I couldn't sustain a normal relationship, and that I would be better on my own. Consequently, our relationship was once more at an end, (the poor man didn't know if he was coming or going). I suggested that Julie come and move in with me. I felt that it would kill two birds with one stone. On the one hand, I would have company and wouldn't need to keep reaching out to men in my desperation. On the other hand, Julie could move out from the oppressive regime at home, and maybe I could help her a bit. Mum and Dad were very reluctant for Julie to move out. They wanted her under their control, and this was especially true for Dad. Anyhow, I managed to persuade them to let her move in with me, with the proviso that she went home regularly to help when they needed it.

I had already asked Alison, the Mind worker, if it would be all right, and she thought that it was a good idea. After Julie moved in, I asked Alison if she would meet Julie, which she did. After she spoke to Julie, I had a private word with Alison. I asked her if she would take Julie on as one of her cases. What she replied shocked me to the core. She said, 'There is nothing I can do for Julie, Susan. In many ways, Julie is far worse than you are. She doesn't even recognise that she has a problem. I would like to help Julie, the fact that she is sharing a flat with you would make that logistically feasible. However, Julie is beyond my help. There is nothing I can do for her.' I knew Julie was in a bad way, but for Alison to say that she was beyond her help, came as a complete shock.

Julie's time with me didn't go very well. We were constantly rowing. I did what I could to help her sort through her bags of religious items. I also tried to help her with her college work, which she had shelved. Her paperwork was in so much mess that she couldn't even lay her hands on anything relevant. I also tried to talk to her about her drink problem, but more often than not, it would end in a row. This was as much my fault as it was Julie's, as we were both sick, and neither of us was in a fit state to have any patience with the other one. In any case, Julie wouldn't accept any help, as she wouldn't admit that there was anything wrong with her. She was living in denial, as the rest of the family were. As I have said before, like the alcoholic, you have to admit that there is a problem before anyone can help you. Julie simply said that she just had to pull herself together.

One evening, Mark, my neighbour, knocked on my door and said that he could hear a woman sobbing outside his flat. I went outside, and to my dismay, I found Julie sitting in her car, crying her eyes out. She had pulled up outside my flat, opened a bottle of wine she had bought, and started drinking. That had obviously triggered the emotions that were now pouring forth from Julie. She must have been sitting there for an hour and a half, sobbing to herself. I said, 'Oh, Julie. Don't sit out here crying. Come into the flat and let me help you. Whatever's wrong, we can sort it.'

I didn't know how I could sort her out. I had trouble sorting myself out. Usually, when she has a few drinks, Julie becomes nasty. The drink releases all the pent up demons inside her. That's what happened on this occasion, and she started verbally attacking me. The essence of the row followed a familiar pattern, that is, I was the root cause of everybody else's problems. All the wrong choices and decisions that I had made, had ruined everyone else's life. No one would even consider their roles in life. It was always my fault.

Because of that argument, I miraculously got Julie to agree to attend an appointment with a GP called Dr. Sutton, (Dr. Gorton had retired by now). I had to beg Julie to keep it quiet from Mum and Dad, because I knew that if they found out, they would cancel it instantly and bring Julie home. I went into the surgery to try to explain to the doctor Julie's problems. However, typical Julie, she kept interrupting me and disagreeing with everything I said. She kept repeating the mantra of having to pull herself together, and that she'd had a bad day but she was all right now. It made me look a real Wally. However, Dr. Sutton was able to see beneath all the camouflage that Julie was attempting to cover the truth with, and she realised that there was indeed a problem.

She said to Julie, 'I think you've got a form of Obsessive Compulsive Disorder.'

Well I knew that she had OCD. I would watch her every evening parking her car and it would take half an hour, walking round and round it, checking and re-checking that the doors were locked. Before that, she would spend 15 minutes inside the car, making sure that everything was switched off. I already knew about her obsessive hand washing, which she did until her hands were raw. However, having Julie living with me made me much more aware of the myriad of problems that plagued her.

Dr. Sutton suggested to Julie that she put her on a course of Amitriptyline, which is a tricyclic antidepressant. It was only going to be a low dose, to bring down the level of anxiety. She said that once the anxiety had been brought down, she could get Julie some treatment for her OCD. She went on to say that until her anxiety was down to a reasonable level, no counselling or psychotherapy would work. Julie agreed, and the doctor wrote out the prescription. I was overjoyed. At last, something was being done about my sister's problems. My problems may well have been insurmountable, but perhaps there was a chance for Julie to overcome hers. We left the surgery clutching the prescription, like the many straws I have clutched at throughout my life.

The next day, Julie was due to go home to Mum and Dad's to run a few errands. I begged her not to say anything to them about her visit to the doctor's, as I knew what the outcome would be if she did. She did tell Mum and Dad. She told them that I had engineered the visit and I persuaded the doctor to put her on an antidepressant. Immediately she told them, they went mad.

They said, 'You see? You've had six weeks living with Susan, and this is the result. She has made you mentally ill. Look at you, you're now on drugs. This is no good. We can't have this. You go back to Susan's flat, pack your bags, and come home right now. You're well when you're here, and you're not well when you're with Susan.'

Julie didn't argue. She came back for her things and left, never to come back. That was the end of Julie getting any treatment for her illness, or even admitting that there was anything wrong. Once again, I was the villain of the piece.

KARL' S BOMBSHELL

When Karl returned to his flat after spending Christmas with Dave and me, he obviously knew that there was no chance of us getting back together as a couple. Because of this, he began ringing chat lines, as I had done a year or two earlier. Now, Karl hadn't told me he was doing this, and indeed why should he? I had my life and he had his; nevertheless, I thought he could have told me as a friend, and I would have supported him.

The first time I suspected something was going on was one evening at his flat. I called there in the afternoon, but I took ill and was unable to go home. The phone rang and Karl looked at me rather sheepishly before answering it. He spoke to the person on the other end in a hushed voice. I could hear bits of the conversation, and heard him say, 'Well, she's still here,' and, 'Yeah, I know, but it's not my fault.'

I realised that the person calling Karl knew who I was, but didn't expect me to still be there. Karl didn't prolong the call, and hung up as soon as he could. He looked very awkward when I asked him who it was, but he wouldn't tell me. He just mumbled something about it being someone I didn't know, and then quickly changed the subject. He later admitted that he used chat lines, but that he only did it to alleviate the boredom. I couldn't blame him, after all, hadn't I done the same thing?

A couple of months later, Karl phoned me and told me that he was going to have a visit from someone that he had met through the chat line.

He said that her name was Sharon and she was a West Indian. He said that she was a mid-wife and she lived in Huddersfield, but she was coming down to London to visit relatives, and would drop in to see him. The day after the meeting, Karl phoned to tell me how it went. He said that they went to a McDonalds, which was a very rare occurrence for Karl. He came in one with Dave and me once. Dave ordered burgers for himself and me, and when he asked Karl what he wanted, he just asked for a coffee.

However, on this date with Sharon, Karl said he had a double cheeseburger with fries and a coke. He said that because this woman was there, he was able to eat like a normal person. The inference was that in that one McDonalds meal, she had cured him. Well, I'm sure that he didn't believe that, and I certainly didn't. I'm not saying that he didn't eat anything in front of her. He once ate a meal in front of Dave, the first time that he met him. If he wanted to impress someone, or pretend that he didn't have a problem, he could do it.

He told me that they were going to get together again in a couple of days, so that he could meet some of her relatives. He said that he would phone me and tell me how it went.

When he called me about that meeting, I couldn't believe what he said. He said that he had been sitting on the sofa, with Sharon feeding him chocolates from a box. He said that this was the woman he had been looking for her all his life and that she had cured him completely of his food problem. I had mixed feelings about all this. If it

was true that Karl's eating problem had been cured by this woman, (which I highly doubted), then I was happy for him. On the other hand, I could see that I was losing him to her.
Logically, I couldn't blame him for looking for someone else. After all, hadn't I done the same thing with Dave? However, since when has love been logical? I still loved him and I still wanted him around me. I suppose that was selfish of me. The rational side of me knew that we couldn't be together and that I should let him get on with his life. However, I was also hurt. I had spent the best part of the last ten years trying to help Karl overcome his problems, to no avail. I had suffered all the crap, lies and deceits, and had bailed him out financially, emotionally and constructively. I gave him everything I had, even when my emotional cupboard was empty. I had gone to hell and back with him, and then in swans this woman and with a click of her fingers, everything was all right. I admit I felt jealous of her, but I also felt bitter. I didn't know this woman and she didn't know me, but she also didn't know Karl. If she thought that it was all going to be plain sailing from now on, she would be in for a rude awakening.

None of this could have come at a worse time for me. I was unwell at the time, not only from the side effects from the medication that I was on, but also with what I was going through with Julie. I hardly saw Karl at all during that period. He had more or less cut himself off from me, and whenever I tried to ring him, his phone was invariably engaged. I should have listened to what David Britten once said to me. He said that when someone else comes along whom Karl could latch on to, he would drop me like a hot potato. I can't deny that I was hurt. I suppose I should have thought, well, I have Dave; Karl has Sharon, let's just get on with our lives. I couldn't. After everything that I had gone through, I suppose I thought that I deserved better.

At Easter, I received quite an elaborate present from Karl. I was surprised, as we never gave each other presents. I knew from experience, that whenever Karl had a guilty conscience about something, he would give me an elaborate present. Soon after, he phoned me from his mobile. He said that he was on a train to Huddersfield to spend a long weekend with Sharon. He said to me, 'You know that you'll always be my soul mate, and you'll always be my best friend.'

Looking back, I realise that he was probably hedging his bets. If it didn't work out with Sharon, he wanted to be sure that I would still be there for him. I said to him, 'Be very careful, Karl. Its one thing her coming down to you, and spending time in a McDonalds. But don't get carried away. Don't commit yourself to anything.'

He said, 'Oh, no, it's all right. I'm only going up for a visit.'

I was worried for him, and I was still looking out for him. However, if I'm being honest now, I was also worried about myself. I still wasn't sure about a life with Dave. The more I thought about Karl and the possibility of losing him, the more I concentrated on his good points. Conversely, the more I thought about Dave, the more I focused on his bad points.

My mind was in turmoil. I wished him luck and said goodbye. I genuinely wanted him to be happy, but I suppose I secretly wanted Sharon to realise Karl's true nature, and end the relationship.

About a week later, I got a phone call from Karl's mum, Kay. She sounded very excited and said, 'I'm about to set off for Huddersfield. Karl is getting married next week.'

I was dumbstruck. Karl getting married? I couldn't believe it.

Kay continued, 'Oh yes, it's very romantic. They had to get a special licence, and they're getting married next Friday in a registry office.'

'What's the rush?' I asked.

'Oh well, they said they knew that they had to get married the first time they met. They love each other very much, but then you knew that didn't you?'

'No, I didn't know that at all,' I said, 'Karl just said that they were only friends. In fact, he's told me precious little about her.'

'Well, you know she's West Indian, don't you?' asked Kay

'Yes, he told me that much,' I said

Kay went on, 'She's been married before, you know. She has a child from that marriage, a little girl of seven. The man she was married to was a bad lot, by all accounts. But this is their chance at happiness. Sharon is very outgoing and exuberant, as is all of her family. It will do Karl a lot of good to be around her.'

Well, I wasn't so sure about that. Karl was the very opposite of exuberant. Kay went on, 'Sharon has an extended family, and they all treat her place as an open house. They're in and out all day. They also have a lot of parties.'

I had to voice my qualms. 'Are you sure Karl can cope with all of that?' I asked. 'After all, the West Indian way of life is completely different to Karl's.'

'Oh no,' she said, 'Karl has completely come out of his shell. Sharon is the best thing that could have happened to him. I wish he could have met her years ago.'

Well, I felt betrayed. After all I had gone through over the last ten years, I was being dismissed. I had been there for Karl through all his problems and I had been there for both Kay and Karl while Tom was dying. I didn't expect Kay to run her future daughter-in-law down, but I did expect a little more loyalty. After all, I always did my best for them, despite having a ball and chain tied to me. Now, Kay was getting excited about this woman who she didn't even know.

Didn't she have any reservations about it? Did I not count at all? I realised that from Karl's point of view, I did the dirty on him, by ringing chat lines, meeting men and then getting serious with Dave. From Karl's point of view, he was well within his rights to do whatever he wanted. I also realised that I had no right to expect Karl to wait in the wings for me to visit him occasionally, while I made a life with Dave. I think that it wouldn't have been so bad if I had been told what was going on. I told Karl at every stage what I was doing. Couldn't he have told me, as the friend I once was?

The night before the wedding, the phone rang in my flat. It was Karl. He said that his mum was there and that Sharon was out. He said that his mum suggested that he ring me. I thought, does it take your mum to remind you to ring me? However, I kept the thought to myself. He told me again that whatever happens, we'd still be friends. He went on to say that since he'd been there, there'd been a party every night.

'What's this Sharon like, Karl?' I asked.

He said, 'She's 27, was a model and she has also been a policewoman. She's now a midwife.' He went on, 'However, we're moving to Gloucester soon, because Sharon's got a new job as a medical rep.'

I thought, 27, model, policewoman, midwife, now medical rep, and married once before, she must get bored pretty quickly. I wondered, perversely, how long it would be before she got bored with Karl. I said nothing.

He went on, 'It's always open house here. There are always masses of people around the place. It's only a three-bedroom terrace, but everyone is in and out of everyone else's room. It's one long party.'

I said to Karl, 'But that's not you. You're like me; you don't like that kind of thing. You're as withdrawn and inhibited as they come.'

He said, 'Oh, but don't you understand. I've come to realise that this is what I've needed all my life.'

The inference was that if I hadn't have been around him, he would have got better sooner. Once more, I was blamed for somebody else's illness. Kay then came on the phone and said that

Karl was eating everything in sight. She said, 'You see Sue, all he needed was the right relationship.'

I felt like I had been punched in the face. I'm sure that he thought I had treated him badly at the end. However, that was due to my illness. I couldn't live with Karl. I didn't have the magic cure that this Sharon seemed to have. I had my own illness to contend with, as well as my dad's and sister's. I was just one person, fighting so many fights, and not winning any of them. I had to put up with a lot from Karl over the years, but I know that it was all down to his illness. I certainly never wanted to hurt him. I loved him, and I wanted the best for him. I always did my best for him. I couldn't have done any more or given any more. Did they not realise this? Did they know how bad I was hurting now?

Karl then had to put the phone down hastily, as Sharon had returned. That made me realise that he either didn't want her to know that he had contacted me, or else she had told him not to contact me. Either way, it certainly put me in my place. I was persona non grata.

Two days after the wedding, the phone again rang in my flat. It was Karl and he was crying. He said that now that he was married, he was going to make a fresh start, and that he was going to cut ties with his former friends that were no longer helpful to him. Apparently, I was one such 'friend' who was no longer helpful. He said that he wouldn't be phoning me again. He was now crying to such an extent that he was unintelligible. Sharon then took the phone from him and said, 'I understand that you're very mentally ill. Obviously, you won't be a good influence to Karl while you're so ill. He can no longer prop you up, as he has done for the last ten years.'

I couldn't believe what I was hearing. Karl propping me up? She went on, 'He needs to get on with his own life now. You can't hold him back any more. So although we feel very sorry for you, we don't feel it's useful being associated with you any more.'

I was sobbing by now, and so unable to answer her. She carried on, 'Karl tells me that you're due to be married to a man called Dave any time now. Maybe he can help you and we hope that it all goes well for you. Obviously Karl's done his best for you, but you have to understand that it's best to cut ties now.'

I didn't know what to say. Yes, it's true that I was ill. This book is testament to that. However, my illness wasn't in the same league as Karl's. Didn't she know that? If you weighed up the help I gave to Karl against the help he gave to me, there would be no contest. It started to dawn on me that Karl was re-writing history. What other lies had been told about me? I was soon to find out.

Sharon said that she would give me one last chance to say goodbye to Karl. He came back on and he was still crying. I managed to get out between the sobs, 'Goodbye Karl. Have a happy life.' I put the phone down and just sat on the floor and cried my eyes out.

About half an hour later, the phone rang again. I leapt up expecting it to be Karl, but it was Sharon again. This time she let loose a tirade of four letter words on me. She said that she had just been on the phone to Kay. She said that Kay told her I made racist remarks about her, and about Karl marrying a black woman. I never said anything of the sort. I just said that the West Indian way of life was completely different from Karl's. She also said that I told Kay that the marriage wouldn't last. Again, I never said that. I merely asked how Karl would cope with an open house, as he was not used to that kind of thing. I was also supposed to have said that they were unsuited to each other. This was all out and out lies. It could only have come from Kay. I thought, this is the final dagger. Kay is turning against me now. How could she, after all I had done for her and her son?

What Sharon came out with next was even more unbelievable. She said that Karl had a lot of credit card and other debts, due to me. 'Don't try to defend yourself,' she said, 'he's told me all about the money you've spent and what you've wasted, and how he's tried to bale you out, time and time again.'

Obviously, she found out about Karl's debts, and he had to try to explain them all away. Instead of coming clean about them, he lied through his teeth. They were my debts and poor old Karl was lumbered with trying to pay them off for me.

She went on, 'I've heard about his flat and the state it is in. You're the reason it's in that state. You didn't lift a finger to clean it. You've done nothing to help him. He's better off without you. You've been a drain on him since the first day you met him.'

This entire outburst was peppered with four letter words. She called me everything under the Sun. She didn't know me, so why was she saying all this to me? It was obvious that it had come from Karl. That's what hurt the most. How could he lie like that? How could he do it to me, after all that we'd been through together? I was so stunned that I could hardly speak, but I managed to say to her, 'You'll find out the truth,' then I put the phone down.

I sat on the floor sobbing. I didn't know what to do. I phoned Dave at his house, and asked him if he would come over. Meanwhile, I looked around my flat. Was Sharon right? Did I live like a pig? Rationally, the answer was an emphatic no. My flat was spotless, because of my cleaning phobia. I kept it immaculate, in order to cut down the cleaning, if that makes sense. I never messed anything up, and that way I wouldn't have to clear up after. That was my coping strategy. However, I was not rational. Part of my illness was to believe anything negative that may be said about me, whether it was true or not. What Sharon said touched a raw nerve. I did have a phobia about cleaning, and worried that I would turn into my Uncle Bernard or my dad. I started dusting and hoovering like a maniac. Dave turned up to find me hoovering the communal corridor outside my flat.

'What's going on?' he asked

'The place is disgusting,' I replied, 'I have to clean it up. Look at all those insects,' I said, pointing to a couple of wood lice. 'I have to get rid of them all.' I carried on in earnest with the Hoover.

I was oblivious to what was going on, because I was having a nervous breakdown. I have been told what happened by Dave and my neighbour, Mark. Dave tried to get me to put the Hoover away, and to go into the flat, so that he could talk to me.

'LEAVE ME ALONE,' I shouted. 'CAN'T YOU SEE HOW FILTHY THE PLACE IS? I HAVE TO CLEAN IT.'

'Come on,' said Dave, 'turn the Hoover off, and then we can talk.'

Dave then unplugged the cleaner, and took hold of my arm, to take me into my flat. 'What are you doing?' I cried in alarm. 'You're trying to kidnap me, aren't you?' I then turned to Mark and said, 'Mark, don't let him take me. I don't want to go to Aylesbury with him. Help me Mark. Don't let him take me away.'

Poor old Mark. What could he do? He liked Dave and he liked me. He didn't want to be in the middle of this. He could see that I was having a breakdown. He said to Dave, 'I don't think you should take Sue away, if she doesn't want to go.'

Dave replied, 'I haven't come to take her anywhere. I've come because she phoned me, because she's having a crisis.'

My head started to clear a bit by now, so I said to Mark, 'It's ok Mark. I have to speak to Dave, but I promise I won't do anything foolish. Thank you for looking out for me.' Dave and I then went into my flat, and I told him all about my phone calls. He agreed with me that it must have been Karl twisting the facts to suit himself. 'Sharon is in for a nasty shock when she realises the truth,' said Dave. 'And if she's as hard as she was on the phone to you, then Karl will also be in for a rude awakening. It doesn't look like he'll be able to twist her around his little finger, the way he did you. But that's their problem now, not yours.'

I had to agree, although I still couldn't get over the fact that I had been stabbed in the back by someone I loved. I could never have done that to him. What was I to do now, I asked myself. I wasn't happy in going to Aylesbury with Dave, but I had Hobson's choice. I knew I couldn't stay in the flat on my own. I couldn't stay anywhere on my own. Going back home to Mum and Dad was out of the question, as well. I just couldn't live in that set-up. I knew that Karl was out of my life forever and I knew that Dave was there for me and that he loved me. If I'm honest, I have to admit that I still didn't love him. I was very fond of him and I knew that he was a good and genuine man, and that with Dave, what you saw was what you got. I knew that I needed someone stable in my life, as I was so unstable. He told me that if I went with him to Aylesbury, he would look after me and cope for me. I believed that he meant it, but did he really know what he was taking on? What if he got fed up with me? Dad said that Dave would come to resent me. Would that happen? Where would I be then? I decided to take a chance. I would go with Dave and set up home with him in Aylesbury. I left Artisan that day. Was I making a mistake? I didn't know. Only time would tell.

LIFE IN AYLESBURY

I moved into Dave's house in Aylesbury. It wasn't easy, as it was quite a small house, and obviously, it was full of all his things. There was no room for my things so I kept everything at my flat in Artisan Crescent. I hadn't yet officially given up my flat, and continued to pay rent there. My family and the social workers were happy about that. They wanted me to keep it, and therefore my independence.

On the other hand, everyone was over the moon about Karl getting married. They thought it was a miracle. As far as Dave was concerned, he had played Karl at his own game and won. He was very happy. I couldn't say the same. I was still waxing and waning over my new life with Dave. One minute I thought that the situation was wrong, and then the next minute I thought that everything would be all right. I was getting pressure from all sides, from people with varying opinions. I didn't know what to do for the best.

The administration at MIND had been patient, but they now wanted a decision from me. If I had left Artisan for good, then they could let my flat out to someone else who would benefit from it. If I was going back, then it had to be now. I had to make a decision.

Dr. Claire Weekes, the notable psychiatrist, succinctly wrote, 'The umbrella has a merry time, going up and down the garden path. Oh that it would rain, so that something outside of myself could make the decision for me.'

That could have been written for me. Normal decision-making was hard for me, to say the least. Having to make a life changing decision was too much. My mind was in a very fragile state. The social workers and my family kept phoning me, pressuring me to keep the flat. Dave kept pressuring me to stay with him, as he said my life was with him now. I couldn't take it any longer. I wanted to be out of this, out of this life and away from all the pressure and entanglement. I ran up the stairs, locked myself in Dave's bathroom, and attempted to take an overdose of my medication and end it all. I didn't even get the packet open before Dave kicked the door in and snatched them out of my hand. I wanted the pain and confusion in my head to stop. I just wanted to fall asleep and never wake up, and then all my troubles would be over. I am thankful now that Dave stopped me, but at the time, I hated him. I had had enough of this life, and all the crap it brought me. I wanted to be out of it, once and for all.

After much deliberation and soul searching, I finally made the decision not to go back to Artisan. Mavis, my social worker, was very angry at my decision. She said that I would have no backup from now on. She said that I had lost her, along with the MIND support.
'I hope you know what you are doing,' she said to me. Me too, I thought.

Well, if I was going to live with Dave, we had to get a bigger place. I needed my things around me, to make me feel more at home. We went house hunting and eventually found a three bedroom mid-terrace in St. Anne's Road. Dave's mum and sister also lived on this estate. Dave said that he would never go back there after he moved out. It was an ex-council estate, and parts of it were quite run down, although the house in St. Anne's Road was exceptionally nice. Dave got a good price for his house, as it was in a prime location, and I put in my 50%. Nevertheless, we didn't have a great deal of money to spend. We could buy either a decent sized house in a less attractive area, or a shoebox in a nice area, which would put us back to square one.

We put in an offer for the house. I felt, naïvely, that if we moved into this big, nicely decorated house with landscaped gardens everything would be all right. My insecurity would go, and I could get on with a normal life. In reality, I shouldn't have been putting in offers for houses. I was not well enough. While we waited for the house conveyed, I had time on my hands at the Pastures while Dave went to work driving his lorry. I began to realize that I couldn't go through with it. I was missing St. Albans, missing my friends and, predominantly, missing my family, albeit that I couldn't live with them. I was also missing Karl dreadfully. I knew he was gone from my life and that I had to get over him, but it was not easy. I was very fond of Dave, and I suppose I did love him to an extent, but he wasn't Karl. If I'm honest, I suppose that I was using Dave as a bolthole. He was secure and safe and an anchor. He was as honest as the day was long, and I knew that he loved me. It wasn't enough. The day before the contracts were due to be signed for the new house, which was a Friday, it all got too much for me. I packed a bag and left.

I didn't know where I was going, but I knew that I had to get out. I just walked to the bus station and got on the first bus. I ended up in Hemel Hempstead and thought, well, what do I do now? I thought that in fairness to the decent, honest, down to earth person that Dave was, I ought to tell him what I'd done so I phoned him on his mobile. I told him that I had run away, and that I was in Hemel. He was distraught. He said that we were supposed to sign the contract for the new house the next day. He was very upset on the phone, and who could blame him. I told him that it was better that we put a stop to the house now, rather than being stuck with something that we would have to sell later on. I put the phone down, as I couldn't speak anymore.

I made my way to a church that I saw as I came in on the bus. I asked to speak to the minister, and someone directed me to his house just up the road. I knocked on the door and a man and woman answered. This was the minister and his wife. They could see how distraught I was, and ushered me into their front room. For the next couple of hours I gave them a potted version of my life. I told them that I had all my savings in the shopping bag that I carried.

The minister said, 'Well, we can't put you up here, but I'll find you a decent homeless hostel that you can go to.'

He then rang round various places, and the nearest hostel that had a vacancy was in Swindon. Later that evening, a member of his church came around, and drove me all the way to

Swindon to a Salvation Army hostel. They took my shopping bag of money and put it in their safe. They gave me a room that had been smashed up by the previous occupant. If that was a decent hostel, it was lucky I didn't get a rough one.

Although it was far from ideal, in a perverse sort of way, the hostel provided a certain safety. Nothing was expected of me and everything was done for me, albeit at a basic level. At least I was free from my constant worry of dust and cleaning. There were two floors at the hostel, one for men and one for women. Some of the residents were long-term occupants. Their rooms were slightly bigger and better than mine, and contained a few of their own belongings. Nevertheless, it was a sad indictment of society that people now called this place home.

One woman was wheelchair bound and suffered from multiple sclerosis. She also had a colostomy bag and had cancer. She couldn't live on her own, because of her disabilities and problems, but had nowhere else to go. She couldn't afford nursing home costs, and so ended up there. The Salvation Army staff were very nice to her, and emptied her colostomy bag and would do shopping for her. Thank goodness for places like that.

Another resident was an anorexic girl, who never spoke to anyone. She was a bundle of nerves, and if you went into the television room and she was there, she would run out. However, because there was nowhere else for her to go, she too was a long term resident.

There was also the usual array of tattooed, drink sodden men and women, drug addicts and the general dross of society. Some would defecate in public places, while others would shout and scream at everyone, and sometimes to nobody at all. Of course, I had come across the same types in various institutions.

The hostel relied on donations of food from supermarkets. The food was not particularly healthy, for instance burgers and the cheapest cuts of fatty bacon and so on. Therefore, you may have a burger, a bit of fried bacon and a slice of fried bread, and that was your dinner. The salt and pepper was chained to the table, along with the sauce bottle. The chairs were similarly bolted to the floor, preventing a drunk or drugged resident smashing up the place. I was quite frightened to go into the dining room, and so I used to go in last, after most people had left. Failing this, I would buy something from the local shops and eat it in my room. At least that way I knew that I was eating something relatively good for me.

I knew that Kay lived in Swindon, and I was quite interested in what had happened to Karl since I last heard. After the way she treated me and lied to Sharon about me, I should have left well alone, but curiosity got the better of me. She was quite nice to me on the phone, and invited me to her flat in the warden-controlled complex. When I got there, she showed me the wedding album. Looking at the photos, I found it hard to understand how Sharon could ever have been a model. I'm not being bitchy, but she really was quite ugly.

I asked how Karl and Sharon were getting on and Kay answered in the positive. She never ran the marriage down, however, she did tell me that Sharon had said to her that she noticed Karl had mood swings and had bouts of depression. Well, he always did, that was part of the illness. Was she starting to find out the truth? I hoped so. Apparently, Sharon talked to Karl about it, and she said that she didn't realise that the relationship between Karl and I was as deep as it was. Sharon merely thought that I was just some friend, a friend who had taken him to the cleaners, by all accounts. However, he said that the split with me was more like a divorce and that he had to have time to get over it. Why should he have to get over it, I thought, who left whom?

Although Kay never ran Sharon down, she did pay me quite a nice complement. She said that Sharon's way was completely different from mine. She said that I was a thorough lady. I inferred from that that Sharon wasn't, but I didn't say anything.

On the Sunday of that weekend, I had to leave the hostel. It was only meant as a stopgap, and that evening the same person that brought me, took me back to the church in Hemel Hempstead. While I was in the hostel, I phoned my friend Kathy and told her what I had done. Kathy and her husband Charlie didn't like the idea of me staying in a hostel and invited me to stay at their house in Bedford. They met me in Hemel and drove me back to their place.

The long-term plan was that the minister was going to try to get me a place in a group home in Rochdale, for people with psychiatric problems. Yet another home. I was grateful for all these people helping me, but what I really wanted was to be well, to be able to cope with a normal life. To have a life. Was that too much to ask? As much as Kathy and Charlie made me welcome, I knew that it wasn't ideal for me to stay there long. I had asked them not to tell anyone where I was. I didn't want the heartache of seeing Dave on the doorstep, asking me to go home with him. However, I missed him terribly. I wanted to hear his voice again, so I phoned him from a phone box to find out how he was. He said that he hadn't cancelled the house, but that he had put it on temporary hold, as he was sure that I would be back. I didn't tell him where I was, but he traced the call to a Bedford call box and it didn't take him long to work out where I was staying.

He came round that evening and put a note through Kathy's letterbox. I watched him walk away, and it broke my heart. I ran out of the house to speak to him, but I was too late. I watched him drive off in his car. My emotions were very unstable and my mind was in turmoil. When he wasn't around I missed him, but when I was with him, I wondered if I could cope with the abrasiveness. It wasn't that he was ever nasty to me or swore at me or even in front of me. It's just that he lived in a male dominated world, (lorry driving) and was used to dealing with rough and ready types day in and day out. Therefore, he spoke more roughly and abrasively than I was used to. He often came across as brusque or crabby, especially when he was in a stressful situation. I found that hard to get used to.

Whenever Dave did a DIY job and it went wrong, he would shout and swear at the hammer that he just banged his thumb with. I know that most men do that, however, I kept thinking that that aggressiveness would be channelled towards me. I had a lot of that from Dad, and I didn't want it again. It never happened with Dave, but that never stopped me thinking that it would. I was also convinced that Dave would get fed up with my illness, and want to end the relationship.

Dad's words to Dave forever echoed in my head. 'You'll resent her. You'll resent her illness. She'll be a millstone around your neck.' I didn't know if that would happen. However, I do know that I couldn't take rejection again. I had all too much of it in my life. I would rather jump than be pushed.

I hope this goes someway to explain my off/on relationship with Dave. It was part of my illness. My mind swung one way then the other. If I had a particularly bad day, my immediate thought was that if I ran away, I would leave my illness behind. Of course, you can't run away from yourself. When you get to your destination, you have to unpack your bags. I had a lot of baggage.

I decided to phone Dave again with a view to meeting up. I told Kathy what I was planning on doing, but she had reservations about it. She knew how unstable I was, and she wasn't sure that I could make any permanent decisions one way or the other. I decided to go ahead, and so I phoned Dave and we agreed to meet in a department store in Bedford. As soon as I clapped eyes on him my heart melted, and I ran to him, kissed him, and held him tight. It couldn't be so wrong if that's how he affected me, could it?

We went back to the Pastures together, and the house sale was back on track, as were Dave and I. For now, at least.

ST. ANNES ROAD

While we were waiting for the house move to take place, Dave and I decided to go on a short holiday to Devon. We stayed in Torquay, and one day Dave suggested that we had afternoon tea in a large hotel called The Grand. Dave was a big fan of Agatha Christie, and he told me that she lived in Torquay and had her honeymoon in this hotel. We sat in the lounge, and ordered tea and scones. Well, the tea came but no scones. We sat and waited and the scones arrived half an hour after the tea, which was now stone cold. To add insult to injury, (as far as Dave was concerned), the scones had currants in, which he hated. So that afternoon we had Dave's version of grumpy old men. The series could have been written for him. All right, the service was slow, and they did bring scones with currants in when we ordered plain, but he moaned non-stop about it. What a miserable git, I thought.

I had an idea of what was coming next. Once everyone had left the lounge, Dave got a ring out of his pocket, went down on one knee, and asked me to marry him. Because I felt for him and I knew that his heart was in the right place, I said yes. His face lit up and I knew how happy he was. My face had a beaming smile on it as well, but inside I felt low and depressed. I wondered how I could live with someone who was so miserable and who hated socialising, when my dream was to be with someone who would give me a social life.

I realise that his attitude that afternoon was because he was nervous and wanted everything to be perfect, but I still hated it. I knew that I was lucky to have a 'normal' man, because I was so screwed up myself. I also knew that he had a big heart and genuinely loved me. Looking deep inside myself, I hated what I saw, as I thought I was a waste of space. I didn't love me, so how could anybody else. I knew that I was not perfect, by a long chalk, so how did I have the right to criticise anyone else?

The day of the move into St. Anne's road came. Dave moved us in his lorry with help from a couple of relatives. Unfortunately, the relatives had to go early, as they had a phone call to say that their little boy had fallen off his bike and had hurt himself. That left Dave and I to carry on alone. As we pulled up outside our new house, the heavens opened. It poured down. Oh great, I thought, just our luck. Anyway, we humped everything inside and sat down for a cup of tea, surrounded by boxes, as you do. I looked around. It really was a lovely house, and I thought that maybe my life would change for the better now. As time went on, however, I began to see why Dave didn't want to return to this estate. Much of it was run down, and quite depressing. Some of the residents left a lot to be desired, as well.

I suppose I had a jaundiced view of the area, as I wasn't happy there. I probably wouldn't have been happy anywhere, as the problem was within me. I didn't know Aylesbury and knew no one there, apart from Mary and Irene. I think that the fact they were literally just around the corner was part of the problem. They were a bit too close for comfort. Of course, Dave didn't recognise that there was a problem. To him, it was the best of both worlds. He had me living with him, with his family nearby. However, it was Dave's family, not mine. My family understood me and my illness, Dave's family didn't, and I didn't have the strength to try to explain.

The problems hadn't gone away, as I knew deep down they wouldn't. The housework problems, the hell of being left on my own, the depression, the fatigue, the battles within my mind; they all continued unabated. Unfortunately, because I couldn't drive and there was no easy public transport route from Aylesbury to St. Albans, I felt cut off from my family. Dave encouraged me to go round to his Mums whenever I felt alone or in need of company, but I knew that wouldn't help. I did Mary's shopping for her, and Dave and I used to do odd jobs around the house and in the garden to try to help them out as best we could. I tried to help them, when I was physically able.

To get me out of the house, and away from the housework, I found myself a job teaching special needs students in Aylesbury College. This was a much-needed outlet for me, and I enjoyed it very much. I also got involved in a prayer group at a local church. Even with all these interests, I still was very unhappy, and one day it all got too much for me, so I packed a case and left. I went once more to stay at Kathy and Charlie's. They had moved to a cottage outside of Bedford, (Dave helped move them), but nice though it was, it was even smaller than their other house. I therefore felt even more of an interloper, and knew that I couldn't stay there long.

When I felt that I had outstayed my welcome at Kathy and Charlie's, I went to stay at Mum and Dad's. It was completely unbearable there, with Dad ranting and raving and telling me that I should go back to Dave. I looked into the possibility of finding a council flat in St. Albans. However, as I wasn't an unmarried mother or a refugee from another country, I had no 'points', and so I had no hope in getting anything.

I also went along to the MIND offices to see if I could get a flat from them. They told me that they were no longer in the business of letting flats, and that anyway, I had a flat once and I chose to leave it. They were quite offish with me, but I couldn't blame them. After all, hadn't I done exactly what they predicted? My only hope was to rent a room privately, which I couldn't afford long term. Anyway, that wouldn't have helped. I knew that I couldn't cope alone, and so living in a seedy room would only make matters worse. I returned to Mum and Dad's feeling dejected.

After a few days, I decided that I had no choice but to go back to Dave. I knew that my mind was not going to get better staying at Mum's, or anywhere else. My problems were inside my head and I had to deal with them. Dave helped me with my fears and phobias. He also pitched in with the housework. I knew that he was my best option for a reasonable life, if he didn't get fed up with me. I decided to go back, even though I hated Aylesbury. For those of you who know Aylesbury and especially those who don't, Aylesbury is a nice town with beautiful surrounding countryside. I just felt trapped there and cut off. You can be anywhere and still be unhappy. Happiness comes from within.

David Hooper

ALL CHANGE

I was at home one day when the phone rang. It was Dave, ringing from the mobile in his lorry. He said that he was sitting in a traffic jam on the M1 and looked out of the window at a railway line next to him. A train flew past him, which put an idea into his head. He said that instead of sitting in traffic jams, he wondered if he could get a job driving trains.

Well, I knew that he was unhappy at his job at Marley Floors; they treated him like dirt and the money was terrible. He had also heard rumours of redundancies, and so he would have to look around for something else, anyway. Consequently, I duly phoned up Chiltern, which was the local railway in Aylesbury, and asked if they took people from 'off the street' to be train drivers and, if so, were there any vacancies. As luck would have it, the woman from the personnel department said that they did occasionally take people from outside the industry, and, in fact, they were recruiting now, but I would have to get his C.V in by the end of the next day to stand a chance. I went round to their offices, picked up an application form, and brought it home. That evening I helped Dave fill in the form and we went round to hand deliver it.

Dave had a good work record and so they asked him for an interview at Marylebone station. He got through the interview and they sent him for a full day of selection tests at London Bridge, which he also passed. Unfortunately, a week or two later, he got a letter back saying that although he had passed all the tests, all the vacancies had been filled by internal applicants. It went on to say that there may be further positions later on in the year. Dave was devastated at this, as we both thought that he was going to get the job. Not to be defeated, however, he asked me if I would ring round to all the other train-operating companies, to see if there were any vacancies anywhere else. With his selection test certificate, he was now a more viable candidate.

The upshot was that he was offered two interviews, one with Virgin in Brighton and one with Thameslink in Bedford. He went along to both interviews and both companies offered him the position of a trainee train driver. It sounds as easy as pie when you read it. However, if you take Thameslink, for example, they only had nine vacancies, but they had over 1500 applicants. If Dave and I knew about all that competition, we may never have gone in for it.

I went along to both interviews with him, and while he was inside being grilled, I went around the estate agents to see about house prices in both areas. As it turned out, we couldn't afford a descent-sized place in Brighton, so we decided against the Virgin job. Another reason for not taking the job was that, although it was a very good company to work for, part of the course meant Dave staying in accommodation in Crewe for six months, while he learned the basics, before being based at Brighton for the rest of the course. Well, I couldn't live on my own for six months and besides, Dave didn't want to live away from home either so he went for the Thameslink post. He said that he had a good feeling about it during the interview, and we could afford a nice place in Bedford. Kathy also lived there and it was on a main route to Mum and Dad's. Things were starting to look up. Maybe there was a God, after all.

Another instance of fate or God having a possible hand in things, was that Dave was offered the Thameslink job on the Thursday, and on the Friday he was made redundant by Marley. He went in that morning, and one of his colleagues in the warehouse tipped him off about what was to happen. Dave took the opportunity to go around the factory to say goodbye to the many friends and colleagues he had made there over the past 22 years. At 9am, the management sent for Dave. He went to the office, knocked on the door and walked in.

'Yes, can I help you?' asked the personnel manager abruptly, barely looking up from behind his desk.

'You asked to see me,' said Dave.

'Who are you?'

'I'm the person whose folder is on the desk next to you.' replied Dave.

'Oh yes, it's Dave, isn't it. Sit down,' said Mr. Personnel. He then handed Dave a letter. 'I think you'd better read this,' he said.

It was a standard 'with regret' redundancy letter. Luckily, Dave knew that it was coming, and so it wasn't a shock.

'So that's it then?' said Dave.

'Yes, that's it. If you go and collect your things from your lorry, I can give you a lift to the station. Have you got enough money on you for your train

fare?' asked this very sensitive personnel manager.
'Yes,' said Dave.
'Good,' said Mr. Personnel, 'let's go then.'
No 'thanks for all your years of hard work', no apologies, nothing.

Mr. Personnel then drove Dave off the premises to the station, as if he was some sort of trespasser. So ended 22 years of loyal, hardworking service. During all that time, Dave had a total of 12 days sick. At the end of it all, the manager didn't even know his name. I almost cried when Dave told me what had happened. However, we had the last laugh. The redundancy money paid for a new car and the cost of the move. Moreover, Dave was moving into a job that paid three times as much as his old one. Even so, I think it was a shabby way to treat any employee, never mind someone who was as dependable and trustworthy as Dave was.

We put St. Anne's road on the market, and we were pleasantly surprised at how much it had gone up in value in the 18 months we lived there. Armed with this knowledge, we set forth to Bedford to do some serious house hunting. It was May by now, and Dave's Thameslink job was to start in September, so we had four months in which to find a house and sells ours. During this time, Dave went to work for a driving agency, and found that he was actually earning more with them than he had at Marley.

We sold our house the first day it went on the market, to the first person that walked through the door, who was a little Indian man and his pregnant wife, both of whom spoke very little English. He offered us the full asking price, and so naturally, we were over the moon. We found a house that we liked in Bedford, and put in an offer. Unfortunately, the vendor pulled out because she became ill and decided not to sell. We started looking again, and found the house of our dreams, (well, at the price we could afford).

The people selling the house, Don and Margaret Coombes, were very nice. We hit it off quite well, and offered them the asking price. We said that it wouldn't be too long before we exchanged contracts, as we had already sold our house to a first time buyer, and therefore there was no chain. We only had to wait for him to get his mortgage together. Unfortunately, the estate agent strung us along about our buyer. They didn't tell us that he was unable to get a mortgage large enough for our house. They kept telling us that he was just undecided which mortgage lender to go with.

This went on for weeks, and the Coombes were naturally getting worried. They had another buyer who wanted the house, and she was willing to pay more for it, in other words, she wanted to gazump us. All power to Don and Margaret, they turned her down, as they said that they wanted their house to go to someone 'nice'. They could easily have sold their house to the woman, and made more money on the deal, but they held off for as long as they could for the sake of us. You don't meet many genuine people like that in the world today, but when you do, it is very refreshing.

One evening, Dave and I were sitting eating our tea and watching Coronation Street, when there was a knock at the door. Dave went to answer it, and it was 'little Indian man', complete with now very pregnant wife and the rest of his extended family. He had a big grin on his face and said in pigeon English, 'I bring my family see house. We come in, yes?'

'Yes, alright then,' said Dave. Well, what could he say? We still wanted him to buy our house. In they all trooped, about ten of them, while 'little Indian man' showed them all around our house. They went in every cupboard and in every room. We felt like we were exhibits in a display. They went upstairs and we could hear laughing. They were all in our bathroom, weighing themselves on our scales. Back they all came, smiling, bowing and thanking us, and Dave showed them out. We were then able to carry on with our tea and telly, still not believing what had just happened.

Weeks went by and we were still waiting to exchange contracts. 'Little Indian man' still had trouble getting a mortgage, and the estate agent was forever telling us that everything would be all right, and that he would be getting the mortgage any day now. The Coombes were getting worried, as they needed a decision soon. They phoned us on a Friday, and said that if the contracts hadn't been exchanged by the following Monday, they would have no choice but to go with the other lady. They said that they wanted us to have the house, but at the end of the day, they needed to know if we could buy it. We went straight round the estate agents and told them outright, that if 'little Indian man' didn't come up with the money by the following day, he had lost the house and we would put it back on the market. It looked like we were going to lose our dream home, but worse than that, we had to go back to Bedford to look for another one. Dave's new job started in 6 weeks and time was running out.

Saturday afternoon, our estate agent phoned us and told us that 'little Indian man' had borrowed the excess from his relatives. The contract was now ready to be exchanged. Dave and I breathed a huge sigh of relief. We got our dream home. The only drawback was that the date of the move was two weeks after Dave started his new job, which meant that he had to drive in from Aylesbury every day, and that the move would come while he had a lot of studying to do. Nevertheless, it couldn't be helped.

As luck would have it, Thameslink have a rest day policy of a 5-day long weekend every three weeks, and Dave's first long weekend coincided with the move. We moved in on the Saturday of the long weekend, helped by Kathy and Charlie, and Kathy's brother-in-law, Frank. At the end of the very long day, we sat once more in a new home surrounded by boxes. But at least we were in, and Dave had three days left of his long weekend to sort the place out a bit.

A month into his training, Dave received a letter from Chiltern, asking if he would like to start there the following Monday. If only we knew. Nevertheless, we were glad we moved to Bedford, especially me. I felt at home there right away. The house was newly decorated with new carpets, so we had to do nothing, which was a blessing considering all the studying Dave had to do at work. The Coombes also left us their new three-piece suite, new wardrobes, dishwasher, everything. They were certainly two of the most genuine people I have ever met. As the Coombes had left us much of their furniture, we were able to sell ours to 'little Indian man', who had none of his own.

Just to round off the story of 'little Indian man', on the day of the move, we had filled the lorry up with all of our things, and so all we had to do was hand the keys over. Well, we waited and waited, but he didn't turn up. We decided to phone him to see how long he was going to be. When he answered the phone, he said in pigeon English, 'I still bed. I come later. You wait two hours.' We couldn't wait ten minutes, let alone two hours, so we told him that he had to come now. He eventually turned up half an hour later, very sleepy, unshaven and unwashed. I've never known anyone so laid back. Anyway, alls well that ends well, as they say.

To cut a very long story short, after a year of hard work, study and numerous exams, Dave qualified as a train driver. I had no idea of what was involved, and in fact, it would make a book on its own. It's certainly more than just pulling a lever, as many people think. I was very proud of him when he qualified, and I like to think that I did my part to help. I helped where I could, by testing him for his rules and traction exams. I tried to support him both emotionally and practically. Dave has supported me during my bad times, and I like to support him as much as I can. I think that's the secret of true love, supporting one another through thick and thin.

KARL UPDATE

I had lost contact with Kay over the years, as I realised that it didn't do me any good raking over the past. Karl was long gone, and my life with Dave, and my love for him, grew stronger by the day. However, for the sake of the book, I wanted an update on his life, so that I could end it properly. To that end, I sent a postcard to Karl via Kay, as I still had her address. She forwarded it to him. I told him in the postcard that I was writing a book about my life and that he featured prominently in it. I asked him if he could tell me how his life was now, so that I could round off the book. I gave him my mobile number, but not my address.

Karl did phone me, and proceeded to give me an update. He asked me if I knew about his daughter, Brittany, whom Sharon had given birth to a year after they got married. I did know that, as Kay told me a few years earlier. Brittany was seven now, he said. He told me that he was no longer married to Sharon. He said that the marriage was very tempestuous, and that he had suffered a lot of physical abuse. In fact, he said that he was a battered husband. I wondered to myself, how long it would take Sharon to realise that I had been telling the truth all the time. If Karl was treating her the same way he treated me, it's not surprising if she lashed out. I knew that she wouldn't be the pushover that I was.

He said that Sharon had more or less led her own life, as a medical rep, and had various relationships along the way. He went on to say that he played the part of househusband during that time, baby-sitting his daughter and stepdaughter. When the little girl was about three years old, Sharon filed for divorce. He had nowhere to go, and so for around a year, Sharon's brother put him up in his house.

During this time, Karl's illness returned with a vengeance. One day, Sharon's eldest daughter went round to visit him and found him collapsed on the floor. He was taken to hospital and from there to an eating disorder clinic. It was a private clinic, as there were no NHS places available. He said that he was very lucky to get in, and that he had very good treatment there. Karl spent about a year in the clinic, and when he came out, he went back to his brother-in-laws' house, while he waited for a council place to become available. He said that while he was at his brother-in-laws' house, he had several catastrophic relationships with unsuitable women that Sharon's brother had fixed him up with. At least, he said that they were unsuitable women. It is more likely that he was unsuitable for them.

He told me that about a year earlier he had a near fatal car crash. He broke both his legs and arms, and cracked a couple of ribs, all of which meant another protracted stay in hospital. He never told me exactly what happened, but he was lucky to be alive. That wasn't the first accident he had, as I have mentioned earlier in the book, but it was very nearly his last. He really shouldn't drive with his illness and addictions.

When I asked him what he was doing now, he told me that during the last year, he had embarked upon an M.A course in Humanities at

Leeds University. He said that he had been able to get on the course by writing a 20,000-word essay, and applied as a mature student. I didn't know that you could do that, but he assured me that you could. Maybe it's true, I don't know. Karl is certainly intelligent enough to do a degree; it's just that after all the lies and deceits he's told me over the years, I'm at the stage now where if he said it was raining, I would have to look out of the window to check.

Karl told me that he now lived in a housing association flat in Huddersfield, and that he still saw his children every day. He picked them up from school and looked after them until Sharon came home. He also told me that he was now engaged to a woman that Sharon had introduced to him in a pub. He said that the woman also had children, and that they were all happy together. I hope it will last, for Karl's sake, but I know from experience that it takes a special person to deal with mental health problems. Most people don't want to know.

That's all I know about Karl's life to date. After speaking to him, I realised that I didn't miss him. Don't get me wrong, there will always be a place in my heart for Karl, and in a way, I still love him. However, the love I have for him now is as you would love an old friend, nothing more. I love Dave, and as time goes on, our love gets stronger and stronger.

As I predicted, Karl's illness is still there, and baring a miracle, will be with him in one form or another, for the rest of his life. I know, because it's the same for me. In fact, it's the same for everyone with chronic mental health problems. They never really go away.

MY LIFE NOW

Well, this is the final chapter of the book, but hopefully, not of my life. That goes on. The illness, too, goes on. Much as I would have liked to end with, 'and so I got better, got a job as a headmistress in a school while standing for mayor of Bedford', that is not real life. This is a biography, not a fairy story. Nevertheless, it's not all doom and gloom. My life has improved dramatically over recent years and the move to Bedford was the best thing I could have done. I felt at home there right away, and my relationship with Dave really took off. We're growing closer together all the time.

I feel that I have taken the rough edges off him and revealed the true person underneath. That person is loving and giving, and has a heart as big as himself. Alison, the MIND caseworker at Artisan, said that is what would happen. She said that he would bring me out of my shell and make me feel wanted and needed, and that in return, I would bring out the soft side in Dave. We both work at our relationship, and our relationship works.

Since I've lived in Bedford, I have been in regular contact with my best friend Kathy, who I love, and I have also made other friends whom I see as often as possible. I have also done some volunteer work as a classroom assistant in a school for kids with behavioural difficulties. It's different from the work I did with the special needs students, as some of the kids can be quite violent, and in fact, some of them have electronic tags attached to their ankles. Dave calls them my 'chained up' class. Nevertheless, I seem to have a way with them, and they do what I ask. I go when I can, although my health problems rear up from time to time, and the chronic fatigue prevents me from doing everything I want. However, since moving to Bedford, I seem to be on a more even keel, and I don't get the black depression and erratic mind changes so much. I've found that I have put Karl behind me once and for all, which means that I can concentrate all my energies into Dave.

When I was young, I used to dream of meeting someone and falling in love with him. It would be a liaison straight out of a Mills and Boon novel. There would be romance, excitement, heart fluttering adoration and fiery passion. I have come to realise that life isn't like that. Many people have started a relationship in that way, only to see it fizzle out over time. With Dave and me, the relationship started out rocky, but ended up bedrock. That is a much better way for things to pan out.

There is a genuine deep love and a solid, long-term commitment between Dave and me. He has taken the time and trouble to find out about my illness, and to help me overcome it where possible. I was on sleeping tablets for 10 years, and I was unable to get to sleep without them. I was addicted to them. With Dave's help, I no longer have to take them. I had the same problem with laxatives. I took them daily to compensate for my overeating. I kept my addiction to them a secret from Dave for years, but once I told him of my problem, he helped me to overcome it.

It's not a nice subject, but I always thought that my bowels would not work properly on their own without the laxatives, as I had been on them for so long, and so I was frightened to come off them. It wasn't easy at first, and in fact, my stomach swelled up to such a size and I was in such pain, that Dave had to take me to casualty. However, I persevered with his help, and now I only take natural ingredients from a health shop. Things are more or less back to normal and 'moving along', as they say.

As for the antidepressants, I do still take them, although they don't cure anything. At best, they take the edge off things. I only take the lowest dose available however, and I go as long as possible without taking anything. I'm not fooling myself or any one else. I'm not cured and I'm far from being out of the woods. My well-being is, in most part, based on Dave's love and care. I know that if I had to live on my own again, all my problems would return with a vengeance. Life is still an uphill struggle for me, and I find it hard to cope with normal day-to-day living. I still have to fight to control my eating, and I don't always succeed. I rely on Dave to help me function, and cope with the housework. On a good day, I can cope quite well. When I get those days, I think that I'm over my problems and I can get on with life. Unfortunately, it doesn't work like that. A few days later, and my fears and phobias return, and I'm back to square one, when again I lean heavily on Dave. Luckily, he doesn't seem to mind. This is a double-edged sword, however. Because I rely so heavily on Dave, I plan my life around him and his shifts. I should be able to function in the house without him, but quite often, I can't.

Sometimes, when I'm having a bad day and Dave's at work, I just have to get out of the house. I would rather get out of the house when the anxiety builds, than turn to food. That just makes me feel worse. I still have thoughts about running away when I get overwhelmed or very unhappy. However, I know that I can't run away from myself. It's like trying to run away from your shadow. My illness goes with me wherever I am, and I have to accept that. I know that my life is with Dave, and that we were meant to be together.

He has written this book, based on my rambling reminiscences, in order to learn as much about mental health problems, and me, as he can. The very writing of the book, and the dredging up of some painful memories, has actually helped me. It was like having therapy, and just being able to see the facts written down in black and white, has helped me to understand why I'm the way I am. I know that my problems haven't been my fault, and that I'm just a product of a set of circumstances. I pray each day to be free from my illness. I don't want to set the world on fire, just to realise some of my potential. I could do so much good, if I wasn't chained to my problems. I have dreams, like anyone, except my dreams are other people's expectations. My dreams are being able to drive, holding down a part time job, being able to cope with housework. It's not too much to ask, is it?

Life at my family home is much the same as it has always been. Since writing this book, my dad has been diagnosed with terminal cancer. He will not get to read this book, and in a way, I'm relieved. I don't want him to see in print that he was the cause of most of my problems. Not that he would ever believe it. As far as he's concerned, he's all right, and it's the rest of us that are crackers.

It is not his fault that I'm the way I am. I blamed him when I was younger, but I have come to realize that he was also a victim of part nurture, part nature, the same as I am, and the same as Julie is. Even though he is coming to the end of his life, the OCPD carries on the same. In fact, if anything, it has got worse. The rules and procedures he implements for every little task have got more and more complex as time has gone on. It goes into every area. This in turn has made life even harder for Dad, as he doesn't have the energy or time to do everything the way he wants it. The result is even more outbursts towards Mum and Julie.

Julie's illness is still being denied by both Mum and Dad, and also by Julie herself. I tried again recently to get her to go a doctor for medication. She refused, saying that she only had to pull herself together. How often have I heard that? The longer she stays in that environment, the worse her condition becomes. I wonder if it's too late to do anything about it now. She is still the sweet natured sister I grew up with, and the nursing care she gives to Dad is invaluable. She also cares for our Aunt Hilda on a regular basis, as she is quite infirm herself now.

That then, is the story of my life so far. It's been far from ordinary or mundane, as I'm sure you'll agree, but I would have given anything for it to have been ordinary. I just wanted to live a normal, boring, life like most people. Instead, I have been shackled with this illness. I'm not feeling sorry for myself, as I have learned to live with it and tailored my life accordingly. I am also fortunate that I found someone to share my life with who understands me and loves me unconditionally.

Dave gives me stability and structure, when my mind is often unstable and the structure seems about to fall around my ears. We enjoy each other's company, and we can talk openly and honestly to one another about any subject. I think that's half the battle, talking through your problems with someone who is willing to listen and cares what you say.

Of course, it works both ways, and I try my best to help and support Dave daily. You have to give and take to make any relationship work, and our relationship works wonderfully. The help and support Dave gives me is invaluable, and his love is unconditional. I honestly believe that God sent him to me. A powerful thing to say, but not said lightly.

'There is no such thing as society,' declared Margaret Thatcher in 1987. I would strongly disagree with that. One of the definitions of society is a group of people living in an ordered community. When Margaret Thatcher's government implemented the Care in the Community policy, a large part of society was broken up. The society made up of vulnerable mentally ill patients.

The basic idea of Care in the Community is a good one. Communities should care for one another. Unlocking the doors of the Victorian asylums and letting people lead a normal life in the community is a sound scheme. For those that can cope, that is. Unfortunately, the Thatcher government did not employ this policy on a purely altruistic basis. It was part of a cost cutting exercise. Close the hospitals and they would save a fortune. However, many feel that it was implemented too quickly, with inappropriate patient selection, and not enough funding for training. In addition, for every success story of a person who thrived after leaving a mental institution, there are a dozen stories of those who couldn't. Of course, patients who were deemed a danger to the public were locked up in secure hospitals. That was necessary to protect members of the public. Nevertheless, many more are in ordinary prisons. Mental institutions are geared to treat mentally ill patients, whereas prisons merely incarcerate.

However, not just dangerous patients are in prison. There are many more are in prison for minor offences, simply because there is nowhere else for them to go. How are they better off? Being mentally ill is not a crime, at least not in this century.

The few sensationalised banner headlines of 'Care in the Community patient attacks man in street', send out a biased view of the norm. People with psychiatric disabilities are far more apt to be victims, rather than perpetrators of crime. Events involving the few, stigmatise the many. Most mentally ill people pose a danger to themselves, rather than to others. For example, around 1000 schizophrenics commit suicide a year, (particularly in prison), compared with 40 murders committed by people with mental health problems.

Sophie Corlett, the Policy Director of Mind said, 'The prison population is increasingly filling up with some of the most vulnerable and socially excluded members of society, and this is having a devastating effect on both individuals and the community as a whole. Mind has argued for years that we need real community services that will identify vulnerable people and offer them support well before the point where they are caught up in the criminal system. There also needs to be a big investment into mental health provision within the criminal system, so that people don't end up in prison when what they really they need is care, and those in prison get the help they need.'

On the same tack, Juliet Lyon, the Director of the Prison Reform Trust said, 'From the moment mental health policy on care in the community disintegrated into a lack of practical support and neglect in the community, hard-pressed prisons began to fill up with petty offenders with complex mental health needs. Proper investment in court diversion, mental health and drug treatment in the community and secure health provision for those who need it, would lift the burden off untrained prison staff and put a stop to the cruel and unnecessary punishment of jailing vulnerable people.'

'Vulnerable people' sums it up perfectly. For many, the community within the mental hospital was all that these patients knew. They could cope in their own small way because they felt 'safe'. As soon as the hospitals started closing, their safety net disappeared. They were placed in complex urban environments, which they just could not cope with. Their institutionalised background made them unable to deal with modern living. In an institution, people can be monitored 24 hours a day. In the community, for the most part, they're on their own.

Obviously, things have progressed over the years. We started with 'Bedlam', then we had 'Madhouses', Lord Shaftsbury gave us asylums, now we have Community Care. Unfortunately, the pendulum has swung too far. There should be a 'halfway house', a sanctuary or refuge for the vulnerable. After all, asylum is just another word for refuge.

I'll climb off my soapbox now. I feel strongly about these matters, as I have worked with vulnerable people half my life, and in fact, I'm one of them. One in four people will be affected by mental health problems in their life. Anyone can get it, at any time. That's a huge percentage, and understandably frightening for anyone who has had no experience in dealing with it. That's one of the main reasons that I have written this book. I wanted to take away some of the taboos associated with mental illness.

It isn't easy explaining what life is like for someone who suffers from mental health problems. If you've never experienced it yourself, then it is like trying to explain colours to a blind man. If, after reading this book, you understand a bit more about the subject, then this has all been worthwhile. Fear and prejudice are based on ignorance. We don't all dress like Napoleon, (who suffered from depression!) or walk around with blood stained axes. We're just ordinary people with various problems.

I'm in good company, however. Some very famous and noble people have suffered mental health problems: Abraham Lincoln, Beethoven, Winston Churchill, Charles Dickens, Isaac Newton, John Keats and Buzz Aldrin, to name but a few.

One of the secrets of dealing with any mental health problem, be it alcoholism, drug addiction or depression, is to acknowledge it and seek professional help as soon as possible. The sooner the diagnosis is made, the more chance you have of overcoming it. I doubt that I will ever overcome my illness. I have had it for so long, and it has so many layers, that baring a miracle, I will have it for life. I have come to terms with that, and thanks to Dave, I am living as normal a life as possible.

As I write this final chapter, I have just found out that Dave has been given the chance to work for Midland Mainline, driving their high-speed intercity trains. It will mean moving to Derby, which I'm in two minds about. Derby is a very nice area and we can get a nice house there. On the other hand, I don't know Derby or anyone there. My friends are in Bedford and so is my volunteer job. I would also be further away from my family at a time when I'm needed. Having said that, Dave has promised that we'll visit home often.

I don't deal with change or upheaval easily and the thought of being further away frightens me. However, Dave is the one with the career. He is very keen to go and I feel that I must support him and give it a try for his sake. Mum has been very positive about it and encouraged us to go for it. Opportunities like this don't happen very often, and as you have read from my life, countless opportunities have passed me by because of my illness. Therefore, I must encourage Dave in this. As I have said before in this book, my problems follow me wherever I go. Nevertheless, with the love of a good man, and the help and support he gives me, I have a fighting chance.

So I have come to the final chapter of the book, but I'm about to turn a new page of my life. Who knows what tomorrow will bring. Whatever happens, knowing me, it won't be mundane.

Susan Kennedy.

Lightning Source UK Ltd.
Milton Keynes UK
UKOW04f0247190615

253726UK00001B/1/P